Intermittent Fasting for Women

The Essential Beginners Guide to Burn Fat, Maximize Weight Loss, Achieve A Lean Body, And Live A Healthy Lifestyle Through Fasting and Autophagy.

Christine Kelly

Table of Contents

Introduction

Welcome to this training manual for Intermittent fasting, your ultimate guide on how to lose fat through fasting.

In this book, you will learn more about the history of intermittent fasting, benefits of intermittent fasting, intermittent fasting and women hormones, kinds of intermittent fasting, what to eat and what to drink while you are intermittent fasting among other useful information.

Chapter One: Origin Of Intermittent Fasting

Definition of Intermittent Fasting

Intermittent fasting is the act of refraining from consuming food for a specified period. Intermittent fasting has two components:

A feeding window- A feeding window is a time interval in which a person is allowed to consume food.

A fasting period- This is a time interval in which a person refrains from consuming food.

Intermittent fasting is not a magic way of losing weight. For instance, you will not lose 10lbs in a week, but you may consistently lose 1 pound every single week.

We can't claim that intermittent fasting is the best way of dieting for every person. It works best for you if you are busy.

Intermittent fasting does not specify which type of foods you should consume, but instead, it determines the time you should eat them. Intermittent fasting is not a diet in the conventional sense, but more of an eating pattern.

History of Intermittent Fasting

Intermittent fasting dates back to the great ancient civilizations. In most parts, ancient civilization such as the ancient Egyptians and the Ancient Greeks were more knowledgeable than you can imagine. Modern scientists are struggling to understand them.

Many written sources are evidence that ancient people used starvation to enable their body to recover and to reap some health benefits that intermittent fasting offered to them.

Regardless of religion or territory, most of the ancient civilization considered using intermittent fasting, and they understood its effectiveness. For instance, Ancient Egypt, Greece, and India are known to have used intermittent fasting to treat some health problems. They also used intermittent fasting as a way of preventing some diseases.

Intermittent fasting was used to strengthen the body as it can kick off processes in the human body. The body can release an organic chemical known as Norepinephrine that functions in the body as a neurotransmitter and a hormone giving you alertness, focus and more energy.

Intermittent fasting also played a significant role in most of the world's religions since it was considered as penitence and self-control.

If you explore the history of different religions in the world and their connection with intermittent fasting, you will discover that people opt for intermittent fasting for various reasons. Judaism has several annual fasting days such as the day of Atonement and Yom Kippur. In Islam, Muslims fast during their holy month of Ramadan. Eastern Orthodox and Roman Catholic have forty days of fasting to symbolize the forty days that Christ fasted in the desert.

In the modern world, scientists are investigating and putting more attention on intermittent fasting. Recent research by scientists from Harvard University shows that intermittent can also increase your lifespan. They found that you manipulate mitochondrial networks inside your cells either by genetic manipulations or by the dietary restriction that mimic it. This could increase your lifespan, and it helps you to improve your health.

Chapter Two: Essential Aspects Of

Intermittent Fasting

Before you browse through different articles about the latest fad diet that can help you to get to your goal of weight loss, you need to note that your aim with any new diet should be how you feel and your health.

Bearing that in mind, intermittent fasting could work well for you if you are smart and more careful with it. Also, you need to be sure that you can go for extended periods without consuming any food.

Your most significant and most essential asset should be knowledge.

Before you opt for intermittent fasting, you need to understand the following aspects.

What Exactly Does Intermittent Fasting Entail?

In this aspect, there are some forms your diet can take. But you need to note that intermittent fasting is the act of restricting the number of calories you can take in 24 hours. You do not cut down the number of calories you have in a single day, but instead, you need to limit the number of hours during the day that you are eating food.

You will fast for about 12 hours, 16 hours or even 20 hours at any given time and restrict consuming food to the remaining 12 hours, 8 hours or 4 hours. Generally, this takes the form of doing away with either the breakfast, lunch or dinner. But you should ensure that you receive your daily calories. There is a more extreme form of intermittent fasting that can be done on a weekly basis. During that time, you need to restrict the number of calories you take to certain hours on some days.

Intermittent Fasting is not for Everyone

Intermittent fasting requires dedication, commitment, discipline, preparation, and knowledge. This is where meal planning becomes very important. Therefore, you need to consider your personality, your culture, and your lifestyle when opting for intermittent fasting. If your body demands food or if you feel hungry after a few hours, then intermittent fasting is not the best for you. Also if you feel like after fasting for about 16 hours you are going to binge for the next 8 hours on cakes, fries, kebab, and a burger, then you will not reap the benefits of intermittent fasting. Your family members eating practices and your schedule may also make an adaption of intermittent fasting a little bit difficult to stick to.

You will also have a challenge sticking to intermittent fasting if you have eating disorders or you have a history of mental illness. Therefore, you need to talk to your doctor before you opt for an intermittent fasting diet. Note that counting the number of calories you consume and going for extended periods without consuming any food can be triggering to you if you are predisposed to taking diet to the extreme. You should be aware that your mental health is as crucial as your physical health.

Intermittent Fasting is not a Quick Way of Dropping a Few Dress Sizes

If you think that using intermittent fasting will help you to drop pounds within a short duration of time because it limits your calorie intake, then you are not going to get the desired results you may wish. To intermittent fasting, you are restricting when you are consuming food, and therefore you should be eating a healthy and the recommended amounts of food. What does that mean then? It means that any amount of visible weight loss may take some time. Note that if you lose lots of weight within a short time on any diet, then it is unlikely that the lost weight will be sustainable in the long run because the extreme restriction is hard to commit to for your life.

Remember that there is no single known miracle diet for a fast and a sustainable weight loss. You should understand that consuming healthy and clean food is what will keep you feel and look your best. Therefore intermittent fasting needs to be your lifestyle that you are committed to if it is going to work well for you.

What you are Consuming is More Important than When you are Consuming it

What the theory of intermittent fasting assumes is that if you are eating three meals a day, you are a bit careful about those meals and their components. Your meal needs to be packed with all the required nutrients you need to survive for the day long, and this is where meal planning comes in. You should be extra careful when planning your meal so that it will contain all the nutrients of vitamins, healthy fats, and proteins. The quality of the food you are consuming when you are on intermittent fasting diet is more important than the hours of the day you are not consuming any food.

It is Possible to Benefit Theoretically Without Fasting

You should try to embrace the theories behind the diet before you attempt the intermittent fasting part. If you are being more careful about the number of calories you are taking to your body, the quality of the food you are consuming and getting all the required nutrients you will have already established a healthier lifestyle. Intermittent fasting is a way to force you to think about the food you are consuming. It is also a way to discourage you from overeating. If you can understand that principle, you can live a healthy life without fasting.

A Moderate Intermittent Fasting Plan Can Work as Well

Twelve hours of starving may sound daunting. But when you factor in 8 hours of sleep, it becomes more manageable. Therefore, you need to establish a moderate intermittent fasting plan that does not involve consciously going for an extended period without eating food. For instance, if you only consume food between 6:00 am and 6:00 pm, you can consume all your meals, but you need to limit late night snacks. Restricting your food consumption to between 9:00 am and 6:00 or 7:00 pm is reasonable for most lifestyles.

Be Smart, Be Careful and Stay Nourished

You need to get all the required calories and macronutrients during the hours that you are allowed to consume food.

Starving your body is not the goal, but your goal is to aim at the quality of food you are eating and to cut out the mindless consumption.

You need to consult your doctor before opting for any extreme meal plan especially if you have other health complications, either physical or mental. Generally, animal studies have concluded that intermittent fasting has a positive impact on blood sugar, but there is no definitive study with human beings yet. If you are suffering from disorders like diabetes, you should talk to your doctor before embarking on intermittent fasting.

Chapter Three: Kinds Of Intermittent Fasting

Intermittent fasting has been the way to go among many women. It can lead to healthy weight loss. It can also improve your metabolic health, and extend your lifespan among other health benefits.

Due to that, several kinds of intermittent fasting has been devised. The different types of intermittent fasting are all effective, but you need to be careful in identifying the one that suits you most.

Ways of Intermittent Fasting

The 16:8 Method: Fasting for 16 Hours Each Day

This method involves fasting for about 14 – 16 hours each day. You restrict your daily consuming window to eight-ten hours. Within the eating window, you cannot fit in two, three or more meals.

The 16:8 method is also known as the Leangains protocol. It was most popularized by fitness expert Martin Berkhan.

Going with this kind of fasting, it can be simple as it involves eating nothing after dinner, and skipping breakfast.

For instance, if you eat your dinner at 8 PM, and then you don't eat until the following day noon, then you have fasted for about 16 hours between the meals.

For women, it is advisable for them to fast for only 14 – 15 hours. This is because women can do better with shorter fasts.

If you are a kind of a woman who gets hungry in the morning and you like taking breakfast, then this kind of fasting is not the best for you. But many of breakfast skippers follow this kind of fasting.

During fasting, you can take coffee, water or other zero-calorie beverages and this can help you to reduce the levels of hunger.

It is crucial to consume healthy meals on your eating window. But note that this will not work well if you consume excessive and large amounts of calories and junk food.

This method of fasting is among the natural ways of doing intermittent fasting. You will put less effort into following it.

The 5:2 Method: Fasting for Two Days in a week

This method involves eating food normally for five days of the week while still restricting the number of calorie intake to between 500 and 600 for the remaining two days of the week.

This type of diet is also famously known as Fast diet. A British journalist Dr. Michael Mosley popularized this type of intermittent fasting.

In this diet, you may choose to eat normally for all days except Tuesdays and Saturdays where you eat small meals with about 250 calories per serving if you are a woman.

Most people find this method of intermittent fasting to be easier to follow and stick to as compared to a traditional calorie restriction meal.

How to Go About the 5:2 Diet

You need to select five days per week when you will normally eat without restricting yourself. The remaining two days you should reduce calorie intake to a ¼ of your daily intake and needs. This translates to approximately 500 calories in a day for women.

Choose any two days of the week you prefer, but make sure there is at least one day in between that you will not fast.

If you eat junk food, you may find yourself gaining more weight. You need to eat the same quantities of foods as if you had not been fasting at all.

If you need to lose weight more effectively, then 5:2 can be the perfect method if you can follow the right procedure. It will help you to consume fewer calories.

It is vital not to compensate for the days you have fasted on much more on the days that you have not fasted.

Eat Stop Eat: Fast for 24 Hours; Maybe Once or Twice Per Week

This method of fasting was popularized by a fitness expert Brad Pilon, and it has become more popular for the last few decades.

It involves fasting from eating dinner to the next dinner. This translates to a total of 24 hours of fasting. For instance, if you consume your dinner on Thursday at 9 pm and you don't eat until Friday at 9 pm, then you will have fasted for a total of

24 hours.

You can also consider fasting from lunch to lunch or from breakfast to breakfast.

Coffee, water and other some noncaloric drinks are allowed during this method of fasting, but you should not consume solid foods.

If your agenda is to lose some weight, then it is vital you consume food in a normal way during the eating period. This means you eat the same quantity of food as if you had not been fasting at all.

The major challenge with this kind of fasting is that a full 24 hours of fasting can be tough for a majority of women to adapt. You can start with 14- 16 hours then you move upwards.

Alternate Day Fasting: Fasting Every Other Single Day

Some of the versions of this method allow you to take about 500 calories during the days that you are fasting.

Many laboratory findings are showing many health benefits if you use these versions of intermittent fasting.

Full fasting every other day may seem to be extreme, and therefore it is not recommended for beginners.

With alternate day fasting, you will be retiring to bed while you are hungry several days in a week. This may not sound pleasant to most people, especially beginners, and it is not sustainable in the long run.

The Warrior Diet: Fasting During the Day But Eating Large quantities of Meals at Night

This kind of diet was most popularized by a fitness expert Mr. Ori Hofmekler. It involves consuming small amounts of vegetables and raw fruits during the day hours and then consume a huge meal during night hours.

Generally, with the warrior diet, you are supposed to fast all day long but feast at night within a four-hour eating window.

Warrior diet was among the first popular meals to include a form of intermittent fasting. This method of fasting emphasizes food selections that are similar to paleo diets: whole and unprocessed foods.

Spontaneous Meal Skipping: This is Skipping Meals When it is Convenient

In this kind of intermittent fasting, you do not need to follow a certain structured routine. You simply skip meals from time to time especially when you do not feel hungry or when you are too busy to eat.

Your body is well equipped so that it can handle more prolonged periods of starvation so missing 1 or 2 meals should not be a challenge to you.

If you are not hungry, you can decide to skip lunch and ensure you eat a healthy dinner. Alternatively, if you are on a trip and you find it hard to get what you want to eat, then you can consider doing a short fast.

Skipping some meals when you are inclined is spontaneous fasting. What you need to do is to eat healthy foods during other meals.

Chapter Four: Mistakes To Avoid On If

If you have decided to try intermittent fasting, you need to save yourself some misery and maximize on the potential benefits by watching out on the following common mistakes.

Binge Eating at Meal Time

When you are hungry, and you sit down to eat some food, it is human nature to overeat because they are suffering from hunger. You need to bear in your mind that overloading yourself with calories will block you from reaping the desirable benefits of intermittent fasting, especially the healthy weight loss.

To lose some pounds of weight, one of the simplest principles to guide you is eating few calories. This means that regardless of the time you are eating, if you are eating the same number of calories or even more than usual you will not lose weight. That is a big mistake most intermittent fasters make. In intermittent fasting, you need to reduce the amount of food you are eating in a day.

Instead of putting a lot of food onto your plate when it is time to eat, you need to portion your diets so that you can know exactly what you are eating and avoid eating too much. If you need some assistance to understand the number of calories to take and the type of macronutrients those calories you are taking should consist, then you can keep a food journal or you can use apps like Fitbit or MyFitnessPal to understand how your food intake matches with your goals and which nutrients you may require more and which you need less.

When you sit down to eat you need to take your time eating

so that your hunger cues will have enough time to kick in and you will know whether you truly need to add more food to your stomach.

Giving up Too Soon

Intermittent fasting is not that easy because you might go all day long on few numbers of calories than normal or sometimes going for long hours than usual without eating food. No matter what kind of intermittent fasting you opt for, the eating style requires you to have high standards of discipline, especially when you feel hungry. You should understand that any feelings of irritability and exhaustion you notice should dissipate after a few days. If they do not, then it is possible that the king of fasting you have opted does not suit your lifestyle and you should reconsider the approach.

Not Eating Enough Food

Most people do not want to undo what they have just done while intermittent fasting for many hours. Some have the mentality that if they eat lots of food the next fasting period may be harder. Consistently eating below your calorie's requirement is a big mistake. It will kick your body into starvation mode thus slowing down your metabolism making it hard to shed fats. So even if you are restricting when eating food, your body still requires enough food so that your organs can function well.

If you feel irritable, weak and unable to focus well when doing intermittent fasting, then it is most likely that you are not taking enough calories. In this case, you can a food tracking application to measure the number of calories you are taking.

Eating the Wrong Food

The moment you do not have many chances to eat food, then what you eat becomes more crucial. Note that it is not just about the number of calories you take, but also the quality of your food. You need to focus on nutrients concentrated foods.

You should focus on eating balanced food with all macronutrients so that your body can function well.

Avoiding Drinking

Many people think that they are not allowed to take anything when they are fasting, but that is not true. Some liquids such as coffee, tea, and water are all good as long you will not add anything like sugar or milk to them. Sometimes you may think that you are suffering from hunger, but in the real sense, you are suffering from thirsty. Therefore, being hydrated may help you during those fast hours.

Forcing it

Do not force intermittent fasting. If you try it and you end up feeling miserable, then you need to re-evaluate to see whether it is the right diet plan for you.

Chapter Five: If And Keto Diets Combined

It is not possible for you to scroll through your social pages without coming across someone talking about the benefits of a keto diet. But if you want keto diet to take you a notch higher regarding weight loss, then you should consider including intermittent fasting to your low carbohydrate meal.

Currently, many people including business personnel, politicians and celebrities are opting for intermittent fasting bandwagon. Keto diet and intermittent fasting work hand in hand to reduce or to accelerate weight loss. They also stimulate other performance benefits in the body. You need to understand that fasting is considered as an extraordinary tool that helps you to improve your biology. Intermittent fasting is adaptable, free and most important it is universal. That is the reason as to why intermittent fasting has always been considered as a significant part of the Bulletproof meal or diet.

Intermittent fasting and keto diet are two distinct dietary strategies, but they have lots of similarities. They both burn fats in the body, and they still boost ketones in the body. When intermittent fasting and keto diet are used together, they are very effective.

You will find most of the keto dieters using these diet strategies simultaneously to accelerate weight loss, increase energy, tackle plateaus and other use them to improve their longevity. They are not causing harm to themselves because these strategies and their benefits have scientifically been proven to be true.

In this chapter, I have explained in details how keto diet and intermittent fasting effectively work together to improve health and to accelerate weight loss. I will also discuss with you how you can incorporate intermittent fasting into your ketogenic diet.

But before we rush there, let me explain to you how intermittent fasting and keto diet work individually.

Ketogenic Diet

The keto diet is a low carbohydrate diet but with a high level of fats. The main purpose of a keto diet is to induce a metabolic state known as ketosis. This is a state where your body stops burning glucose, but instead, it burns fats to produce energy.

The reason as to why your body burns fats is the fact that there is the absence of glucose that could provide energy to your body cells and also produce ketones that your body uses to fuel your brain and other major organs in the body.

Ketones are some water-soluble molecules that replace glucose in your body when carbohydrate intake is insufficient.

The main benefit of a ketogenic diet is weight loss, but other benefits may include but not limited to improved energy, mental clarity, cancer prevention, improvement in neurological disorders, diabetes control, hormonal balance and reduction of cholesterol.

Initially, the ketogenic diet was designed to treat epilepsy disorder among the children. This idea was developed back in the 1920s. Before then researchers found that a meal with low carbohydrate and high level of fats led to the elevation of ketones.

After a few decades, researchers found that keto meals provided benefits that are beyond the control of epilepsy. Today, wellness enthusiasts in the whole world are embracing and encouraging the consumption of a ketogenic diet. But most of them are using the keto diet to control diabetes and boosting weight loss. After all, you need to remember that a keto diet is a low carbs diet with a high component of fats.

Several studies indicate that a low carbohydrate, high-fat diets like keto meals are the most effective for the loss of weight as compared to a low-fat diet or a classic calories reduction.

These diets are more natural to adapt because they suppress appetite.

Intermittent Fasting

This kind of diet is more concerned about when to eat rather than what to eat. In other words, it is a diet that is based on the timing of food consumption, but it is not based on restricting calories intake and eating a specific type of food. In this dietary strategy, you eat and fast within specified windows of time. For example, doing away with breakfast and taking your next meal during lunch time or dinner constitutes intermittent fasting.

There are distinct types of intermittent fasting, but in this book, we will discuss only three common types. They include;

Skipping of Meals

We have already mentioned it in our previous section. It is a scenario where you skip any meal as you may wish. You may prefer skipping either breakfast, lunch or dinner.

Eating Windows

This strategy is the most popular approach to intermittent fasting. It restricts food consumption during specified consumption windows. Some people prefer specified windows with numbers such as 16:8 which means 16 hours of fasting and 8 hours of consumption windows.

Alternate Days Fasting

This strategy involves fasting for some few days of the week and consuming regular meals in the other days of the week. People consider this strategy as the most difficult of intermittent fasting.

The main goal of intermittent fasting is to reduce the quantity of food you consume in a day. When you consume food, you can only eat small quantities of food. When you restrict your feeding windows, you will consume less food than you could do with more meals a day.

Why Intermittent Fasting Works?

Different cultures and religions in the world have been fasting for many decades as an alternative medicine for millennia as well as spiritual practices. Fasting has been prescribed as a treatment option because it can treat almost every health condition.

Recently, researchers who were examining the positive effects of fasting concluded that occasional fasting is good for human beings. Moreover, researches have shown that calories restriction, for instance during fasting is one of the proven approaches that can make you live longer.

And when mentioning calories restriction, this is one of the main reason why fasting works. You should note that overeating causes high cholesterol, diabetes, obesity, and some heart disorders. All these diseases are a threat to the world today. Fasting works well because it has been proven to cause significant changes in the biochemical and metabolism processes on the cellular level.

How Intermittent Fasting Works

Remember that when you consume more food than what your body requires to produce energy, your pancreas releases a chemical known as insulin. The insulin generated signals the body's fat cells to store calories for later use. The opposite of this process will happen if you do not consume anything. The insulin levels in your body will decrease, and this leads your fat cells to release some of the stored fats in your body. What I mean is that fasting directs your body to use the stored fats to produce energy.

Human body exists in 2 metabolic states, fasted and fed. The fasted metabolic state is when the glucose levels are deficient while the fed metabolic state is when the levels of glucose in the blood are high. Glucose levels in the body drop or rise depending on the amount of carbohydrate you consume. The reason behind it is that your body is used to run on glucose but not on protein or fat.

Apart from accelerating weight loss and fat burning, intermittent fasting is effective in improving the overall health of human beings. This is because when fasting, your cells are under stress. Therefore the cells respond to the stress by enhancing their ability to resist diseases.

Why Keto and Intermittent Fasting?

Keto diet and intermittent fasting affect the metabolism states in the same way. That is they both cause ketosis. I know you are asking yourself; Then why not just use either keto or intermittent fasting? The answer is that intermittent fasting may be a bit difficult when you are not on the keto meal plan. Also, the ketogenic diet is boosted with intermittent fasting.

As a keto dieter and you have already entered ketosis, you will have low levels of glucose in your body cells. Also, insulin levels are in full burning state. You will also have a reduced appetite because of the satiating effects of a ketogenic meal. Ketone levels will also be elevated in your body cells. This goes without saying that you will experience no sugar crashes and you will be less hunger when you are fasting.

When you have opted for the standard high carbohydrate meal, and you do not eat for an extended period, the glucose levels will drop in your body, and you will experience a rise in the hunger hormones. If this happens, you may experience irritation, weak and shaky.

Chapter Six: Intermittent Fasting And

Metabolic Change

Body fats are the only way to store calories or energy in your body. When you do not consume anything, your body changes several activities to make the stored calories more accessible. These changes may occur in your nervous system as well as in your essential hormones.

Here I have listed some of the several changes that may take place in your metabolic system when you fast.

Insulin- When you consume food, insulin level in your body increases and when you fast, the insulin level in your body decreases. When the insulin level is low, it facilitates your body to burn fats.

Human Growth Hormone- Growth hormones are essential hormones in the body because they aid muscle gain and loss of fats. Changes in the level of growth hormones can skyrocket during fasting. It can increase as much as 5- fold.

Norepinephrine- During fasting, your nervous system sends norepinephrine hormone to your fat cells thereby making them break down body fats into fatty acids which are later burnt to produce calories.

Studies show that fasting for 48 hours may boost your metabolism by about 3.6- 14 percent. On the other hand, long periods of fasting may suppress your metabolism.

How does Intermittent Fasting Help You to Lose Weight?

One of the primary reasons that this kind of fasting works well for weight loss is that it will help you to eat fewer calories.

Several protocols involve skipping some meals during fasting periods. Not unless you compensate by consuming much more during the period of eating, then it means you will be consuming fewer calories.

According to a recent study that was conducted back in the year 2014, intermittent fasting can help you to lose weight. According to this research, intermittent fasting was proved to reduce weight by about 3- 8 percent within a duration of 3- 24 weeks.

When investigating the rate at which people lose weight, it was found that they lost about 0.25 kilograms within a period of one week when they were on intermittent fasting, but they lost 0.75 kilograms with alternate day fasting within the same period of one week.

Women were also seen to lose 4-7 percent of their waist circumference. This indicated that they lost some belly fats.

These findings and conclusions are impressing, and they indicate that intermittent fasting is a useful method of losing weight.

All said and done, the advantages of intermittent fasting go far beyond just weight loss. Intermittent fasting has other numerous benefits such preventing chronic disorders, metabolic health and it can as well expand your lifespan.

Generally, calorie counting is necessary when you are on intermittent fasting, but in most cases, weight loss is mediated by a reduction in calories intake. Researchers comparing continues calorie restriction, and intermittent fasting indicates that there is no difference in weight loss when calories are matched between groups.

Intermittent Fasting May Assist You to Hold on to Your Muscles When Dieting

The major side effect intermittent dieting is that your body will tend to burn fats as well as muscles. But interestingly, some researches indicate that intermittent fasting can be beneficial for holding on to your muscles when you are losing your body fats.

In one review research, intermittent calorie restriction was seen to cause similar amounts of weight loss as that of continuous calories limitation. But this happened with a smaller reduction in the body muscle mass.

During the calories restriction findings, 25 percent of the weight loss was body muscle mass as compared to about 10 percent in the intermittent calories restriction research.

One of the studies had participants eat the same amounts of calories as there before, except one huge meal during the evening hours. It was found that they lost their body fats while increasing their body muscle mass along with other health benefits.

Intermittent Fasting Makes Healthy Eating More Simpler

One major benefit of intermittent fasting is its simplicity. For instance, instead of eating more than three meals per day, you can eat two meals, and this makes it easier to maintain your lifestyle.

A single but best diet for you is a diet that you can stick to for an extended period. Therefore if intermittent fasting is the easiest for you to stick to a healthier diet, then it will have long term health benefits and weight control.

How to Succeed With Intermittent Fasting

For you to lose weight with intermittent fasting, there are some things that you need to bear in mind.

The quality of food- Note that the type of food you consume is still essential. You need to consume a whole and single ingredient type of foods.

Calories- They still count. You need to eat normally when you are not fasting, but you should not consider compensating for the calories that you missed when you were fasting.

Consistency- As you could do with any other method of weight loss, you have to stick with intermittent fasting for an extended period if you want intermittent fasting to work for you.

Patience- Note that intermittent fasting may take extensive time for your body to adapt. Therefore, you need to be consistent with your meal schedule, and this will work well with you.

Popular intermittent fasting procedures, recommend extensive strength training. It is very vital when you want to burn your body fats while still holding on to your body muscles.

Note that, in the beginning, counting calories is not necessary with intermittent fasting, but if the weight loss stalls, then calorie counting becomes a useful tool.

Generally, intermittent fasting can be a vital tool to lose body weight. A reduction in calories intake primarily causes it, but there are beneficial effects on hormonal that comes into play.

Chapter Seven: Benefits Of If

The main benefit of intermittent fasting is weight loss. However, there are several benefits of intermittent fasting, and most of them were widely recognized even in history.

In ancient times, fasting periods and seasons were referred to as cleanses, purifications or detoxifications, but the idea of all of them is the same. That is to do without eating food for a specified period. Ancient people believed that this period of fasting would clear their body systems of any toxin and rejuvenate them.

Some of the most known benefits of intermittent fasting are;

Improved Mental Concentration and Clarity

Fasting has incredible benefits for the healthy function of the brain. The most known benefit stems from the activation of autophagy, which is a cell cleansing process. Note that fasting has anti-seizure effects.

Since the time immemorial human beings have been known to respond to caloric deprivation with a reduced size of major organs with two exemptions, the male testicles, and the brain.

This preservation of testicle size is a significant benefit because it helps to pass on genes to the next generation.

This preservation of cognitive functions is essential for the survival of any human being.

For instance, imagine you are a caveman where food is scarce.

When your brain starts to slow down the mental fog will make it harder to get food. Your brain power, one of the major advantages you have in the natural world, could be decreasing. Surviving without food will slowly erode your mental functioning until you are a slobbering idiot. You will be incapable of essential blundering functions let alone going out to get or to hunt food.

Therefore, for survival, cognitive functions in your body are maintained and boosted during fasting or starvation.

This aspect has been known throughout the evolution of humankind. For instance, in ancient Greece, thinkers or scientists used to fast for days.

They fasted not because they wanted to lose some weight. They believed fasting would increase and improve their mental agility. Even today, people marvel at the ancient Greek mathematicians and philosophers. Even in the history of Japanese prisoners during the Second World War people have been describing the unquestionable clarity of thought that accompanies starvation and fasting. This book describes a prisoner who would read several books from his memory and another prisoner who mastered the Norwegian language in a few days.

Mental Sharpness and Intermittent Fasting

Consider and think about the large Thanksgiving turkey and pumpkin pie. After that meal, were you mentally sharp? Or were you dull? What about the opposite when you were hungry? Were you slothful and tired? The answer is a big no. When you were hungry, your senses were hyper-alert, and your mind was very sharp. The fact that consuming food would make you concentrate even better is not true. There are survival advantages to human beings that are cognitively sharp. You will also experience physical agility when you are fasting.

Research has found that mental acuity increases with fasting. One of the studies compared cognitive task at the bottom line, and after 24 hours of fasting, they found that none of the mentioned tasks including attention focus, sustained attention or simple reaction time was found to have been impaired. In addition to that study, another double-blinded research of two days caloric deprivation found that there were no detrimental effects even after several testing for cognitive performance, sleep, mood, and activity.

When you say that you are hungry for something, such as hungry for attention, hungry for power, does it mean that you are dull and slothful? It does not mean that. It means that your mind is energetic and hyper-vigilant. Hunger and fasting activate you toward your goal. Many people tend to think that fasting would dull their senses, but the truth is that it has an energizing effect.

Therefore, there will be an increase in your brain connectivity and some new neuron growth in your stem cells. This is mediated in part by your brain-derived neurotrophic factor. For women, both fasting and exercise increase brain-derived neurotrophic factor expression in many parts of their brain. BDNF plays a major role in glucose metabolism, appetite, and control of gastrointestinal and cardiovascular systems.

Intermittent Fasting & Neurodegenerative Disorders

There is also another aspect of neurodegenerative diseases and fasting. If you maintain intermittent fasting, you will experience less age-related deterioration of neurons as compared to a person who is on a normal diet. You will also experience fewer symptoms in diseases such as Huntington's, Parkinson's, and Alzheimer's disease.

The benefits of intermittent fasting to your brain can be experienced in both during caloric restriction and fasting. During calorie restriction and exercise, you will experience increased electrical and synaptic activity in your brain.

Neurogenesis is a process in which stem cells differentiate themselves into neurons that are capable of growing to form synapses in the absence of other neurons. Note that both calorie restriction and exercise increase neurogenesis through pathways such as BDNF.

Moreover, the level of fasting insulin appears to have a direct inverse relationship to your memory as well. This means that when you can drive down your fasting insulin, you will experience improved memory score.

If you have increased body fats, which can be measured through Body Mass Index, it will lead to a decline in your mental abilities. If you measure your blood flow to the brain, you will find that a higher Body Mass Index is linked to a decreased blood flow to some areas of the brain that are involved in higher function, reasoning, and attention.

Intermittent fasting is among the perfect methods to decrease insulin while still reducing the number of calories intake.

Intermittent Fasting and Alzheimer's Disorders

These complications are characterized by an abnormal accumulation of proteins in the body cells. There are two classes of Alzheimer's disorders, that is neurofibrillary tangles and amyloid plaques. The known symptoms of Alzheimer's disorders closely correlate with the accumulation of these tangles and plagues. These abnormal protein accumulations in the body cells are believed to negatively affect the synaptic connections in your memory and the cognition parts of your brain.

Some specific proteins such as HSP-70 are known to prevent damages and misfolding of amyloid and neurofibrillary tangles proteins. Therefore alternate fasting will increase the levels of HSP-70 protein. When amyloid and tau proteins are destroyed beyond repair, they are removed by autophagy. This process is also accelerated by intermittent fasting.

Risks of Alzheimer's disorders are related to obesity. Recent research found that abnormal weight gain in middle ages predisposes to Alzheimer's complications.

When taken together, it implies a possible fascine in preventing Alzheimer's disorders. Over 6 million of the American population have Alzheimer's disorders, and this may even increase further due to the aging population. Alzheimer's disorders create huge burdens to family members who are forced to take good care of their affected members.

Intermittent fasting has lots of benefits in reducing weight, type 2 diabetes and its complications such as kidney disease, heart attacks, cancer, strokes, eye damage, and nerve damage. Moreover, the possibility exists that intermittent fasting prevents the development of Alzheimer's disorders as well.

The method of prevention may also affect the autophagy. This is a cell self-cleansing procedure that enables your body to remove damaged proteins from your brain and the body at large.

Since Alzheimer's disorders result from the abnormal accumulation of amyloid and tau proteins, intermittent fasting provides an opportunity in which your body cells can get rid of the abnormal proteins.

Intermittent Fasting and Breast Cancer

Low-calorie meals are a strategy to prevent breast cancer. It has beneficial effects on the overall health of breast cells within the breasts of a woman. Overweight women have large fat cells in their breasts, and this increases the amount of estrogen within the breast. They can also store fats in their liver and in their abdomen where it increases the circulation of sex hormones, insulin hormone, inflammation and fat produced hormones. These changes in the liver and the breast leads to the development of breast cancer.

Therefore eating low-calorie diets will reduce the fats in the abdomen and the liver. This will reduce the levels of insulin hormone hence reducing the risk of breast cancer development.

Intermittent Fasting and Insulin Sensitivity

As far as metabolism of glucose is concerned, intermittent fasting is perfect. It is a powerful tool that normalizes glucose.

It also improves the glucose variability.

Weight Loss

Note that intermittent fasting is an effective way to lose some weight if you can do it properly. Regular short-term fasting can allow you to consume less number of calories.

Several types of research reveal that intermittent fasting is as a perfect weight loss tool as the traditional calories restricted meals for short-term weight loss.

A recent review of studies in the year 2018 in overweight adults revealed that fasting led to weight loss of about 6.8 kilograms within 3 – 12 months.

Another study found that intermittent fasting can reduce body weight by 4 – 8 percent of obese women within a period of 3 – 24 weeks. The same review also revealed that an adult woman could reduce her waist circumference by 4 – 7 percent within the same period of 3 – 24 weeks.

You need to note that long term effects of fasting on weight loss for adult women remain to be seen.

Note that in the short-term, intermittent fasting appears to aid in weight loss for women. But the amount of the weight you lose is dependent on the number of calories you eat during the periods that you are not fasting. It also depends on how you adhere to your lifestyle.

Intermittent Fasting and Eating Habits

Ideally, opting for intermittent fasting will naturally help you to consume less food.

Research in 24 hours healthy women was concerned at the effects of long 36 hours of fasting on consumption habits. Apart from taking more calories on the fast post period, women who participated decreased their total calories balance by about 1900 calories which were a significant decline.

Chapter Eight: Side Effects Of If

In our previous episode, we have talked about the major benefits of intermittent fasting. You need to give it a try, but at the same time, you need to understand some side effects of intermittent fasting that you may experience during your journey of intermittent fasting. Remember that your body requires some time to acclimate to any extreme change. Therefore you will experience some notable side effects when you stop consuming food for an extended period. In the beginning, these side effects can be unbearable, but if you can understand how you can deal with them you will be able to continue with your intermittent fasting and later on, you will reap all the benefits of intermittent fasting.

As a woman, before opting for any new meal plan including keto diet, intermittent fasting, and other meal plans, you need to consult your doctor for advice.

Some of the common side effects of intermittent fasting are;

Hunger

When you are used to consuming lots of food several times in a day, your body will expect to be fed with food at certain times. Note that your body has a ghrelin hormone that is responsible for making you feel hungry. This hormone peaks mostly at dinner, lunch and breakfast time and it is generally regulated by food consumption. When you start fasting, the levels of ghrelin hormones will continue to peak, and you will suffer from hunger. In the beginning, it will take serious willpower. You may experience the worst from day one to day five, but after that, it will reach a time when you will not feel hungry.

If you want to combat hunger during the first week of your intermittent fasting, you need to drink lots of water. This will help you to keep your stomach full, and you will not feel hungry. It will also help you to stay alert. It will also satiate that feeling of having to consume something. Therefore within 45 minutes after you wake up in the morning, drink at least one liter of water. In the day if you feel hungry take another one liter of pure water. You can even drink more than one liter; it will not harm you. One important thing that intermittent fasting will teach you is that what you thought was hunger may be boredom or thirst.

Drinking tea or black coffee can help you to combat hunger as well. Also, keep yourself busy and active, get enough sleep, and avoid strenuous workouts at the beginning, since that can lead you to feel hungrier. Consuming enough food the day before is another perfect way of preventing hunger.

Cravings

If you consume a slice of orange, again and again, the chances are that what you will want to do is to eat a slice of orange. During intermittent fasting, you will have extended periods without eating. So you will think about eating now and then. That is when the aspect of cravings kick in. You will find yourself yearning for refined carbohydrates and sweets because your body is trying to look for that glucose hit.

What you need to do is to do anything you can do but never think about food. Be sure to indulge a little bit during the feeding window so that you can have a chance to satisfy your cravings.

Headaches

As your body is not used to fasting, you will experience dull headaches that will come and go. Dehydration can be a major cause of abnormal troubles. Drink lots of water during both your feeding windows and fasting time.

Moreover, headaches can be caused by a decline in the level of blood sugar or by a stress hormone that is released by your brain when you are fasting. As time goes by, your body will become used to fasting, but it is essential you try as much as possible to avoid stress.

Low Energy

Remember that during fasting, your body will no longer be getting the exact source of energy it used to get from consuming food. Therefore you will feel sluggish at the beginning. To avoid this, keep your day relaxed, and as much as you can, exert the least amount of energy. You should give your workouts a short break, or you just perform light exercises such as yoga or walking. Also, consider sleeping for more hours.

Irritability

Note that the feeling of hunger is real and to some extent, it sucks.Avoid circumstances that may annoy you and consider focusing on performing activities that will make you happier.

Bloating, Constipation and Heartburn

Remember that your body produces some acid that helps you to digest food. So when you are not consuming food, you will experience heartburn. But this side effect is not common as compared to others. It could range from mild discomfort to burping for extended hours. This condition will be cured with time but ensure you drink lots of water. Also, prop yourself up when you are sleeping. When you eat, avoid spicy and greasy food that can exacerbate heartburn.

In addition to heartburn, intermittent fasting can cause constipation which can cause discomfort and bloat. To avoid constipation during intermittent fasting, drink lots of water.

Feeling Cold

During intermittent fasting, you will experience cold toes and fingers. Why do you feel cold? When you are fasting, the blood flow increases to the fat store cells. This will help your body to move fats to the muscles where it will be burnt to produce energy. When the level of glucose decreases in your body, it can make you feel cold. You can prevent feeling cold by drinking hot coffee, wearing extra layers, taking warm showers and more importantly, avoid going outside for extended periods when it is cold.

Overeating

Sometimes you feel so famished when your fasting window comes to an end that you tend to eat fast and later end up consuming more food than you would. When your fasting period is over, be mindful about your diet. In some cases, you may want to reach for a slice of pizza, but it is a good idea if you can go for the grilled chicken instead.

Regular Bathroom Trips

Remember that during intermittent fasting, you will be drinking tons of water to stay hydrated. Due to that, you will be forced to visit the bathroom regularly. You can even find yourself visiting the bathroom thrice per hour. This is a side effect you can not avoid, and therefore make sure you are always near a washroom.

When to Quit?

All the above side effects sound bad, but they only last for a few days. The best way to alleviate the above side effects is to ease into intermittent fasting. Do not go from consuming five meals in a day to consuming two meals. Just give your body time, and intermittent fasting will become more natural and healthier, with more mental sharpness, and less appetite in the long run.

Listen to Your Body

Intermittent fasting is not meant for everyone. For instance, pregnant and nursing mothers, women with diabetes among others should not opt for intermittent fasting. If you are managing a chronic disorder, you should always seek doctor's advice before you opt for any new meal plan. Also if you have a history for developing eating disorders, you should avoid intermittent fasting of any kind.

There comes a time when the above side effects should not be ignored. Intermittent fasting is not meant for you if you feel dizziness because of low levels of blood glucose, if intermittent fasting is interfering with your ability to be responsible, or if you find yourself developing an unhealthy obsession with food. You need to cut your fasting short and consume food earlier than your planned time. You may also consider stopping fasting altogether. When you experience any strange issues, it is always good to seek doctor's advice.

Chapter Nine: Why If Is Better Than Other Diets

I believe you must have come across many books telling you what you should be eating and how best you can lose weight. Ideally, there are low carbohydrate diets, intermittent fasting diets, paleo diets any many more types of diets. But which among the diets is the best for sustainable and effective for weight loss and even good health?

To start, let us look at low carbohydrate diets such as Dukan, pioppi, and Atkins. The argument behind them is that carbs are bad for health because they are broken down into sugar which in turn stimulates the release of the insulin hormone. The insulin helps your body to store the energy from food as fats around your middles.

What is not argued in this discussion is that not only do carbs encourage your body to make the insulin hormone but also food with a high concentration of fats and protein do this as well.

Related to low carbohydrate diets are evolutionary approaches such as paleo and caveman diets. These types of diets recommend shunning the processed food, and you have to follow a diet that is similar to what ancestors used to eat during the Paleolithic period.

Description of this type of the diet can vary, but they tend to exclude most grains which generally results Than low carbs diet. You should also avoid dairy products in this diet. Both paleo and low carbohydrate diets recommend you eat lots of fresh food like vegetables and little-processed food.

Low carbohydrate diets may help you to lose weight, reduce your risk of heart disease and even reduce the risk of type 2 diabetes. However, these benefits are mostly linked to the energy restriction, they cause and are not directly related to avoidance of carbs.

Weight loss: Healthy body weight loss requires low levels of caloric intake and intermittent fasting does it automatically. The reason as to why weight loss diets work is the fact that they reduce the number of calories you take.

This implies that your body will be burning more calories than you take leading to weight loss. And intermittent fasting is not an exemption to this rule.

Skipping some of your meals reduces the number of calories you take, and therefore you do not need to worry about the level of calories in the food you eat.

Unlike other diets, intermittent fasting will help you to lose the actual fats: When you want to lose weight, I believe you actually want to lose body fat and not your muscle mass or much water. Intermittent fasting will help you to lose less muscle mass and more fat mass as compared to other low-calorie diets and detoxes.

Intermittent fasting will help you to preserve muscle mass that may be lost with other diets: Note that most weight loss meals can cause you to lose fats and muscles which may become a big problem. To maintain your muscle is essential to make sure your metabolic rate does not go down.

Intermittent fasting is useful when you gain the holiday's weight: As we have seen that weight gain in the human body occurs gradually over many years or even decades. Minimizing holiday's weight gain each and every year will help you reduce some pounds of weight.

Chapter Ten: The Science Behind If

The Theory Behind Intermittent Fasting

For several decades, scientists have been arguing that intermittent fasting makes evolutionary sense. It can be true because since the genus homo evolvement over two million years ago people were hunters and gatherers. When people went to the forest and successfully hunted an animal, it meant that they were to have two or three days of feasting on a diet that was rich in calories(meat). But when the feast was over, they fed themselves with low-calorie roots, berries, and cereals.

In turn, that led over many years to metabolic or biochemical adaptation. This was through a natural selection process that maximized the survival capacity in those uncertain food supply circumstances.

Remember that our protein, fat and carbohydrate metabolic pathways are similar to the metabolic pathways of bonobos, gorillas, and chimps, who are our close relatives who did not adapt to intermittent variations of calories supply.

There are important adaptations that impact the results of intermittent fasting. Intermittent fasting lowers your metabolic rate precisely. This is because your metabolism is structured in such a way that it can conserve energy that is related to the uneven supply of calories in the body.

The challenge is that it works in the opposite direction of the people opting for intermittent fasting to burn a greater number of calories.

On its face, it is a challenge to invoke the aspect of hunter-gatherers paradigm. For more than ten thousand years when the man invented agriculture, the supply of calories has been in plenty and predictable. People have not lost their metabolic adaptation of energy conservation, but they got progressively plumper and recently even obese.

What does this mean physiologically? It means that the human's metabolic setpoint is higher as compared to the ancient times of hunting and gathering and the hormones are geared to maintain physiological stability that will resist any change in the metabolic set point which we are all aware of.

There is also another complex information when it comes to the metabolism theory of hunters and gatherers. It is believed that gut flora plays a vital role in the metabolic fate of macronutrients. Note that obesity can cause a radical change in the gut flora. Moreover, the new gut flora may promote further obesity. Maybe hunters and gatherers did not have this challenge.

Scientific Evidence

The problem of intermittent fasting was first employed by Panda and his colleagues from the Salk Institute. Most of the human body functions are controlled by a master pacemaker that is situated in the brain structure known as the suprachiasmatic nucleus.

The pacemaker gets a neutral signal from your eyes, and therefore it is primarily controlled by the light and the dark periods. Note that in a similar arrangement to your federal system, every organ in your body has its sub-pacemaker that is designed to serve the particular requirement of that specific organ.

In his research, when he withdrew food from mice for 24 hours period, he found that about 90 percent of the genes in the liver that were under the circadian regulation of the clock stopped to function. It is not surprising because we would expect the major metabolism organs to be controlled by the supply of food.

On the other hand, we can let the mice consume a high-fat diet for 24 hours in a day, and you will find that all the genes that are under the control of the liver circadian pacemaker getting activated around the clock. What came is that the mice became obese, and this explained the mechanism of fasting and feasting on the molecular level. To answer the question about the benefits of intermittent fasting on human beings, there is no well know substitute in humans.

The Human Experience

Among the most consistent pioneers of intermittent fasting for weight loss is a nutritional researcher Dr. Krysta Varady from the University of Illinois in Chicago. The lady published widely and deeply on the subject matter, and she summarized her findings in a book, *The Every Other Day Diet*. Her book had a tagline of "4 weeks, two sizes, 12 pounds." Dr. Krysta Varady also ran an important experiment before her conclusion.

In a magazine entitled JAMA that has been published recently, Dr. Varady reported of research that was carried out of one hundred obese people. These participants included 86 women and 14 gentlemen. These people were randomized to three different groups for one year: alternate day fasting (25 percent of energy needs on fasting days; 125 percent of energy needs on alternating feasting days), calorie restriction (75 percent of energy needs every day) or a non- intervention control.

The research was carried out for six months of weight loss phase that was followed by a six months weight maintenance phase.

In addition to the groups being randomized and professionally controlled, the trial lasted for one year, unlike other short-terms studies.

Results

Intermittent fasting is tricking your body and mind into consuming less food. And because you are losing weight, you are benefiting from the metabolism. This implies better compliance through mind tricks although Dr. Varady concluded that the study did not produce superior adherence.

Nevertheless, there is much to admire in Dr. Varady here. She is a researcher who devoted her time and career to proving the clear benefits of intermittent fasting. She dared to run the definitive experiment. She also had the intellectual integrity to explain the facts, however inconvenient it looked.

Intermittent Fasting & Autophagy

Definition of Autophagy

The word autophagy was derived from Greek words *auto* meaning self and *phagein* which means to eat. Typically, the word autophagy implies to eat oneself. This is a body's mechanism when your body gets rid of broken down and old cell machineries such as proteins, cell membranes, and organelles. It happens when there is insufficient energy to sustain them. This process is regulated to recycle and regrade cellular components.

Another known process is apoptosis or programmed cell death. Your body cells are programmed to die after some division. In the beginning, this process may sound kind of macabre, but it is a good process for your health. For instance, imagine you have a motor vehicle. You love this motor vehicle, and you always have great memories of your motor vehicle.

But after a couple of years, your motor vehicle starts to get beat up. Given another few years, your motor vehicle is not looking great anymore. Therefore, your car will cost you some dollars every year to service and maintain it so that it can look good. It is knocking all the time. It is, therefore, a wise idea to dispose of it and buy a new model car.

That is similar to what happens in your body. It reaches a time when your body cells become old, useless, and junky. That is the reason they are programmed to die the moment their valuable time is over. This may sound cruel, but that is how life is. It is similar to leasing a car, where after a specific period of time you will get rid of the vehicle regardless of whether the vehicle is in excellent condition or not. Then you consider getting a new car.

Autophagy Replacing the Old Parts of the Cells

As the case with your car, it also happens at subcells level. In this case, you do not need to replace your entire motor vehicle. In the specific circumstance, maybe you only need to replace the tire or the battery, and you throw away the old one and replace it with a new one. This is exactly what happens in your body cells. Rather than killing off the whole cell, a process known as apoptosis, you need to replace some parts of the cells. That is the process of autophagy.

In the autophagy process, subcellular organelles are destroyed, and new ones are rebuilt to replace them. Note that organelles, old cell membranes, and cellular debris can be removed. This process can be done sending it to a specialized organ called lysosome that contains enzymes that is responsible for degrading proteins in the body.

Autophagy process was initially described back in the year 1962 when several researchers found an increase in the number of lysosomes in the liver cells of a rat after they infused glucagon. Christian de Duve, a Nobel-winning scientist, is the one who came up with the term autophagy process. In the autophagy process, the damaged parts of cells and the remaining proteins are taken to the lysosomes to wind up the job.

The main regulator of autophagy is a kinase known as mammalian target of rapamycin. When this kinase is activated, it tends to suppress autophagy, but when it is dormant, it promotes the autophagy process.

What Accelerates Autophagy?

The major activator of autophagy is the deprivation of the nutrients in the body. Note that glucagon is an opposite hormone to insulin. It is like the game that kids like playing called opposite day. When glucagon goes down, the insulin goes up. Therefore, as you eat food, glucagon tends to go down, and the level of insulin rises. The rising level of glucagon accelerates the process of autophagy. Fasting raises the level of glucagon in your body, and this is a much-known activator of autophagy.

This is cellular cleansing. Your body identifies substandard and old cells and marks them for destruction. Note that the accumulation of all these unwanted cells is the one responsible for many known effects of aging.

Intermittent fasting does two critical things. First, by stimulating autophagy, you will be clearing out all your old, junky cellular proteins and some cellular parts. Secondly, fasting stimulates growth hormone that directs your body to produce new snazzy parts for your body. You will be giving your body a complete renovation.

Note that you should get rid of all old and unwanted stuff before you can consider putting in new stuff. For instance, think about renovating your house. If you have an old crappy 1950's style cabinets hanging around, you need to dispose of it before buying and installing a new one. The process of destruction is as important as the process of creation. It will not make any sense if you try to put in a new cabinet without removing the old one.

Intermittent fasting may reverse the aging process because it helps you get rid of damaged and old cells and replacing them with new cells.

Autophagy as a Highly Controlled Process

This process is highly regulated. Note that if it runs out of control it will be detrimental and therefore it must be controlled. In your cells, the total depletion of the amino acids is a signal for autophagy, but the work of the individual amino acids is more significant and variable. However, you need to note that the level of plasma amino acids varies only a little bit. Insulin signals and amino acid signals converge on the mTOR pathway. This pathway is also known as the master regulator of nutrient signaling.

Therefore what happens during autophagy is that unwanted old junk cells are broken down into the amino acids. I know you are asking yourself ''what will happen to these amino acids?'' During the early stages of fasting and starvation, the levels of amino acids go up. It is believed that these amino acids that are deprived of autophagy are delivered to your liver for gluconeogenesis. Also, these amino acids can be broken down into sugar or glucose through the tricarboxylic cycle. Another important fate of the amino acids is to be incorporated into new protein cells.

The negative consequence of old junky protein accumulation in the body can be witnessed in two main disorders, that is cancer and Alzheimer's complications. Note that Alzheimer's disorder is caused by the accumulation of abnormal proteins either tau or amyloid proteins which may gum up your brain system. Therefore autophagy is a perfect process because it can clear out some old protein cells and it can prevent the development of Alzheimer's disorder.

What turns off the autophagy process? It can be turned off by eating. Therefore insulin, glucose and proteins, all of them can turn off autophagy. And to turn it off, it does not matter how much you take. Even a small amount of amino acids can stop the autophagy process. Therefore the autophagy process is unique to fasting, and in most cases, it can be found in simple diets or caloric restrictions.

This is where there is a balance. You get sick from too little autophagy as well as from too much autophagy. This gets you back the natural cycle of life- fasting and feasting where there is no constant dieting. Note that life is all about balance and nothing else.

Fasting as a Self Destruct

Ironically for people who cleanse their body by drinking tons of juice, eating actually has been proved to work against the autophagy process. For many people skipping meals is a stressful activity that their bodies may not immediately love but it has incredible benefits.

Studies have proved that there are lots of benefits to seasonal fasting and some of these benefits such as heart diseases and the risk of diabetes may be accounted to autophagy.

Fasting accelerates and promotes autophagy in the brain. Therefore it is an effective way that helps to lower the risk of neurodegenerative disorders such as Parkinson's and Alzheimer's.

In other studies, intermittent fasting has been known to improve brain structure, neuroplasticity and cognitive function that may help your brain to learn more efficiently. All said and done it was not clear if the autophagy process was the root cause, plus those studies were done on rodents and not on human beings.

Benefits of Autophagy

It May Save Your Life

Note that autophagy is an ancient mechanism that its main function is to preserve life. In times of infection, stress, and starvation, the process of autophagy kicks in order to maximize repair while still minimizing damage. Combining intermittent fasting with fats as a source of energy while activating autophagy concurrently can starve an infectious intruder of sugar and reduce inflammation so that your immune system will have an easier time repairing damages caused by inflammation and infection.

Autophagy Reduces the Risk of Neurogenerative Disorders

Most disorders of aging brains take too long to develop because they are; as a result proteins that are around the brain cells that do not work right. The autophagy process helps your cells to clean up the protein components that are not performing their tasks, and therefore they are less likely to accumulate. For example, in Parkinson's autophagy removes synuclein and in Alzheimer's disorder autophagy removes amyloid.

Autophagy Assists you to Regulate Inflammation

Autophagy process promotes the amount of inflammation by assisting to boost your immune system. It can increase inflammation when an invader enters your body by triggering the immune system to attack.

It helps you fight the infectious diseases

Autophagy helps recruit an immune response when required. Moreover the process of autophagy removes certain microbes like viruses and mycobacterium tuberculosis from the inside of cells. It can also remove the toxins that are created by infections.

As you create inflame and microtears muscles during exercises, your muscles will require repair. The demand for energy will increase. The cells of your muscles will respond to this by the autophagy process so that they can reduce the amount of energy required to degrade the damaged components and to improve the balancing of energy to reduce future damage.

NB: Autophagy process is among the most important breakthroughs when it comes to the science of aging. Though this process has been known since the early 1950s, it is only in the last few decades that scientists have been able to see the benefits of activating autophagy to improve the health of human cells. In our previous section, we have learned how autophagy can enhance and promote your cell maintenance by removing unwanted and damaged cells and by using recycled components as a nutrient resource. This implies that the autophagy process promotes longevity because an organism can recover quickly from stress-induced cellular damage. When your body cells are effectively able to clean up the damaged cells, it implies that they will perform their functions better.

Chapter Eleven: What To Eat When Fasting

Though the term fasting sounds scary, intermittent fasting is taking the world of weight loss by storm with recent research on the IF's positive impact on individuals' body weight, blood pressure, and cognition.

It is no surprise that your friends and relatives are jumping on the intermittent fasting bandwagon. But maybe the appeal is the lack of food rules and regulations. There are some restrictions on when you can consume food, but not necessarily about what you can consume. Therefore should you be consuming bags of chips and pints of ice cream while intermittent fasting? NO. That is why in this book I have listed the best food that you need to include in your intermittent fasting lifestyle.

Intermittent Fasting for Beginners

Here is a little but helpful information to new beginners of intermittent fasting diet. Remember that there are multiple intermittent fasting plans, but most of them focus on doing away with food for a certain duration of hours in a day, days or even for weeks.

There are no restrictions or specifications about how much food or what type of food you are supposed to consume while you are on intermittent fasting. But the benefits of intermittent fasting are not likely to accompany consistent diets or meals of big macs.

A well-balanced meal is a key to healthily losing pounds of

weight, maintaining the levels of energy and sticking with the meal plan. Therefore if you are focusing on losing weight, then you need to focus on macronutrients- dense food such as fruits, whole grains, beans, nuts, veggies, seeds as well as lean proteins and dairy products.

How to Schedule Your Meals

Before you opt for an intermittent fasting meal plan, it is essential you talk to your doctor to ensure that this is right for you. Ladies should be more cautious because there are mixed opinions on whether or not some intermittent fasting protocols are healthy for the development and balance of the female hormones.

If you are suffering from adrenal fatigue or you have gut health complications, you can proceed with the intermittent fasting but with caution. But if you have a history with eating disorders, then you should avoid intermittent fasting altogether.

The moment you start your intermittent fasting journey, you will most likely feel fuller for an extended period, and this can keep the food you consume very simple.

What to Eat During Intermittent Fasting

Avocado

It may appear counterintuitive to consume the highest calorie fruits while trying to lose some pounds of weight, but the monounsaturated fats found in the avocado fruits are incredibly satiating. Several types of research have concluded that even adding a quarter of an avocado fruit to your lunch meal can keep your stomach full for many hours.

Fish

There is a reason the dietary guidelines suggest consuming at least 8 ounces of fish per week. Fish is not only rich in healthy proteins and fats, but it also contains a good amount of vitamin D.

Cruciferous Veggies

These are food like brussels sprouts, cauliflower, and broccoli. They are full of fiber. The moment you are eating erratically, it is important you eat food that are rich in fiber to prevent constipation. In addition to that, fiber can make your stomach feel full for an extended period, which is something you may wish to experience if you can not eat again for about 16 hours.

Potatoes

Initially, potatoes were considered to be bad, but you need to note that not all white potatoes are bad. Potatoes are among the most satiating food around. Consuming potatoes as part of your healthy meal can help with your weight loss. But note that potato chips and French fries do not count.

Legumes and Beans

The favorite addition to your chilli may be your best friend on the intermittent lifestyle. Carbohydrates supply energy to your body for activity. But note that I am not telling you to carb-load, it definitely would not hurt to throw a few low-calorie carbohydrates such as legumes and beans into your meal plan. Black beans, lentils, chickpeas, and peas have been proved to decrease weight even without restricting the number of calorie intake.

Probiotics

Do you know what the little critters in your gut like most? Diversity and consistency. That implies that they are not happy when they are hungry. When your gut is not happy, you will experience irritating side effects such as constipation. To deal with this unpleasantness, you need to add probiotic-rich food such as kefir, kraut or kombucha to your meal plan. The farmhouse culture referred to as Gut Shots are perfectly known for any 500 calorie days because each 1.5-ounce shot may brim with live 10 billion CFUs for just ten calories.

Berries

Your favorite smoothie addition is ripe with essential vitamins. Note that berries like strawberries are good sources of immune-boosting vitamin C. It has more than 100 % of the daily value in a single cup. That is not even the best part because recent research found that individuals who consumed any diet rich in flavonoids such as strawberries and blueberries had smaller increases in body mass index throughout 14 years as compared to those who did not consume berries.

Eggs

A single large egg has six grams of protein, and it cooks within minutes. Note that during your intermittent fasting, you need as many proteins as possible so that you can build muscles as well as to keep your body full. A recent study concluded that women who ate eggs for breakfast instead of eating bagels were less hungry and they ate less throughout the day. What I mean by saying this is that when you are looking for something to do during your fasting hours, you need to boil some eggs hard.

Nuts

Nuts may be higher in calories as compared to other snacks, but the advantage is that they contain good fats that other junk food do not have. Scientists suggest that the polyunsaturated fats that are found in walnuts can alter the physiological markers for satiety and hunger.

A 2012 research study found that one ounce serving of 23 nuts has 20 fewer calories than what is listed on the label. Generally, the chewing process doesn't completely break down the nut cell walls. It leaves a portion of the nut somehow intact and unabsorbed during the digestion process.

Whole Grains

Being in a certain diet and consuming carbohydrates seem like they belong to 2 distinct buckets, but that is not always the case. Remember that whole grains are very rich in proteins and fiber and therefore consuming some goes a long way in keeping your stomach full. Remember that consuming whole grain items instead of the refined grains may rev up your metabolism. Therefore during intermittent fasting, you need to consume whole grains. Venture out of your comfort zone and try amaranth, bulgur, millet, and farro.

What to Drink during Intermittent Fasting

Water

Though you are not consuming food during intermittent fasting, you should hydrate your body due to many reasons. Note that good health is a major organ in your body. The amount of water that you should take varies — dark yellow urine indicates that you are dehydrated and it can cause fatigue, lightheadedness, and headaches.

Intermittent fasting may take different forms, but all of them require taking water. Avoiding water for many hours is dangerous to your health. It is essential you remain hydrated when you are intermittent fasting. Dehydration can lead to mood changes, kidney stones, constipation, and unclear thinking.

If there is some food intake that is involved during intermittent fasting, for instance, 500 calories per day on calorie restricted periods, then it is recommended you take about nine glasses of water.

When food intake is restricted in any day during intermittent fasting, more of the hydration will come from plain water.

Generally, women are advised to take about 11 glasses of

water. You can stay hydrated if only you let thirst to be your guide.

Coffee and Tea

While fasting, you can take coffee and tea. When your intermittent fasting calls for zero energy intake, then you will not add sugar, milk or cream to your beverages. Therefore you should drink them plain. A recent study that was conducted in the year 2018 on intermittent fasting allowed unsweetened herbal teas and black coffee.

The moment you are taking caffeinated tea and coffee which may have a mild diuretic effect, then ensure you balance them out with pure water. Decaffeinated teas and coffee ensure that you are going to get the hydration effects that are needed from your beverage.

Juices

Juices are not calorie-free, and they will not fit in with a no-calorie intermittent fasting plan. However, nutrients during intermittent fasting are essential. Fasting sounds like you are not going to eat or drink anything, but several types of research on intermittent fasting include some calories on the fasting days.

In fact, 100 percent juice is a perfect way to provide your body with nutrients and energy during fasting, but it should be integrated into low-calorie food. From that aspect, high water, low-calorie food such as celery, lettuce and watermelon may be satisfying because they will give you a high volume of food per calorie.

Other Drinks that are Suitable for Intermittent Fasting

One of the drinks you need to consider during intermittent fasting is fruit infused water. This drink is hydrating, and it can keep the palate more interested in fasting periods. You can infuse your drinking water with either oranges, mint or strawberries.

Another perfect drink is unsweetened almond milk. This drink tends to be low in calories. It is fortified with vitamin D and calcium.

In addition to the above drinks, you can take warm, savory clear broths because they can help you to make a low calories meal feel more satisfying. For instance, you can take chicken, beef or vegetable broth.

Intermittent Fasting and Vegetarians

Vegetarians avoid eating meat as much as possible either due many reasons, whether that is health issues, taste preferences, or they simply do not agree with the fact of eating animals. These people are not exempted from intermittent fasting and like any other person, they will reap the benefits of intermittent fasting if they follow it carefully.

Here are some of the foods that vegetarians can eat during intermittent fasting.

Sweet and sour pineapple sticky rice

For you to succeed in intermittent fasting, you need to

discipline yourself. It is essential you fill your eating time frame with balanced and nutritional foods. This is most important for vegetarians, who mostly rely on plant-based diets.

Among the best ways to meet your satiety is by knowing what makes food filling. Note that filling food items contain high levels of fiber, water, and protein. They also have low energy density. You should, therefore, eat foods that are high in those ingredients and ensure you are taking water frequently.

Whole grains

Incorporating whole grains into your diet is a perfect way to keep your belly full for an extended duration of time. Whole grains will keep all your parts of the kernel such as germ, endosperm, and bran. Note that your body tends to digest the whole grains at a slower rate and therefore you will remain full for long.

To start your day, take a bowl of porridge or oatmeal. Oats are a good source of fiber, and they have low levels of calories. You can incorporate the oat with seeds and nuts. After some few hours, or later in the day, you can eat Persephone bowl, mushroom and kale farrow, roasted beet sorghum salad or buckwheat poori.

Vegetables with starch

Starchy vegetables are heavier and robust. They include white and sweet potatoes, pumpkin, beets, carrots, winter squash, and corn. These vegetables may keep your belly full for an extended period but be careful not to overdo them because they contain high levels of carbs. Being carbs, starchy vegetables have high levels of glucose as well, which can be difficult for your body to break.

As a vegetarian, you need to try foods like winter squash and sage pizza, or butternut squash hash browns.

Nuts and Seeds

Seeds and nuts are perfect additives for a meal. They also offer a hearty snack for vegetarians. Therefore, you need to sprinkle them on your crush and consider roasting them in squash dishes. They contain fiber and proteins that will help your stomach to remain full for a long duration of time. They also have unsaturated fats to help stabilize the levels of insulin.

In vegetable recipes, nuts will offer a savory and buttery alternative ingredient for dairy-free cheese and toppings. On the other hand, seeds pack a punch of nutrients.

Legumes

Note that legumes are plant-based diets because of their versatility. They are alternative to meat when it comes to the aspect of satiating. Legumes are high in protein and fiber while they contain low levels of calories. Lentils are one of the most common legume, and you need to have them in your vegan kitchen.

Chapter Twelve: If And Loss Of Weight

You will find that many weight loss diets have lots of complexities and rules. But intermittent fasting tends to keep things simple. In fact, for the last few decades, intermittent fasting has become a common eating habit of losing weight among many women.

Weight loss requires a deficit in calorie intake

This is mostly achieved through intermittent fasting because intermittent fasting does this automatically. Remember that we have said that the reason weight loss diet works are it reduces the number of calories you consume. This implies that you will be burning a greater number of calories than you consume and this will lead to a loss of weight.

Intermittent fasting is not exempted from this rule. When you skip either breakfast, lunch or dinner, it greatly reduces the number of calories you consume. Therefore you do not need to worry about the number of calories in the meal you consume. For instance, you will have saved about 500 calories every day by skipping a breakfast of orange juice or peanut butter toast, as well as whatever you might drink or eat for morning tea.

Given the average lady might be aiming for 1600-1800 calories in a day to lose weight, that will be a whopping 30 percent of the number of calories saved instantly.

If you skip the morning meal, even indulging in 2 large 750 calorie meals some hours later in that day, plus 300 calories dessert which will total to 1800 calories, will keep you on track for your weight loss.

Note that weight loss is all about consuming fewer calories than you burn. If you miss even one meal per day, you can save about 30 percent of calories at a go.

Intermittent Fasting Will Help you to Lose Actual Fats

Unlike other diets, intermittent fasting will help you to lose the actual fats. I believe when you say that you want to lose weight, you mean that you want to lose fat.

Typically, you do not wish to lose your muscle mass. Studies indicate that intermittent fasting will help you to lose more fat mass and less muscle mass as compared to very low-calorie meals or weight loss detoxes and cleanses.

This study showed that intermittent fasting helped women to cut 4 – 7 percent of their waist circumference within 24 weeks. This implies that they lost their actual belly fats which are harmful fats around the organs. These studies and conclusions are in line with a recent review that looked at all the current evidence.

The studies found that as compared to opting for a very low-calorie diet, for instance, less than 800 calories, alternate day fasting causes about 8.4lb or 3.8 kilograms extra fat loss.

With Intermittent Fasting, You May Preserve More Muscle Mass than you Can Lose When Dieting

There is a big problem with other weight loss diets because they cause you to lose both fat and your muscle.

Maintaining your muscle is essential to ensure your metabolic rate does not drop and to support a healthier weight loss.

If you fail to do that it means that any fat loss will come back fast. This is what happens typically with any biggest loser contestant.

Intermittent fasting is more useful than the regular calorie restriction for overweight patients since it leads to better preservation of your muscle and more significant loss of body fats.

Another researcher found that 25 percent of weight loss was muscle mass in a normal calorie restriction meal as compared to just 10 percent in intermittent fasting calorie restriction meals.

High protein diets and weight training are essential aspects of maintaining and building muscle mass. Therefore if you want to try intermittent fasting, make sure each of the food you consume has a source of quality proteins such as meat, fish, legumes or eggs.

Note that intermittent fasting can help you to preserve your muscle while still losing fat. But this must be coupled with proteins intake and resistance exercise.

Intermittent Fasting is Helpful When you Gain the Most Weight

Typically, weight gain occurs gradually over many years or even decades. But note that the amount of weight you gain in a single year is not consistent though. It spikes over the Christmas and Thanksgiving holidays.

In fact, the period between November and January is responsible for about 50 percent of the weight gained within 12 months.

Therefore if you can minimize Christmas and Thanksgiving

holidays weight gain every year, it will go a long way on the scales of weight loss.

The major challenge is following a restrictive meal during holidays because it means you will have to track macronutrients and calories. Otherwise, you may miss out on all the good things.

My advice is straightforward. If you are invited for a substantial lunch by your friend or a relative, you should skip breakfast entirely. You can even consider consuming a light dinner the day before.

You can also decide to miss a meal or even two meals the day after feasting. In that way, you do not have to miss out on your favorite treats.

Remember we have said that most women gain weight during the festive season. Intermittent fasting is an eating pattern that helps you to minimize the number of calories you consume, but it allows you to enjoy your holiday feasts without any restriction. **Intermittent Fasting does not Cause Yo-Yo Dieting**

Yo-Yo dieting refers to the cyclical gain and loss of weight over a given period.

Consider Restrictive diets like water fasting, detoxes and cleanses, and low-calorie meals.

Twenty-four hours is not enough period for severe calorie restriction to kick your appetite hormones into overdrive. When intermittent fasting is broken up into intervals, it does not cause the yo-yo effects. Intermittent fasting cuts down the number of calories without a major impact on the feeling of your hunger.

Note that a single day of severe calorie restriction is not good enough to negatively affect your hunger hormones that are what occurs during yo – yo meals.

How will intermittent Fasting Help You Lose Weight?

When you are fasting your body will use its stored body fats to produce energy. Burning calories in this way will help you not only to lose some weight but also any excess fats in your body that you may be carrying. This implies that you will not be just thinner, but you will also look better and healthier.

Intermittent fasting can help you to optimize the release of fat burning hormones in the body. These hormones are insulin and the growth hormones.

How Much Weight Will You Lose?

The amount of weight you may lose with intermittent fasting will be determined by how regularly and how long your fasting periods are, and more importantly what you eat after fasting. For instance fasting for about 16 – 20 hours each day will help you lose about 2 – 3 pound of fats each week.

Chapter Thirteen: If And Your Lifespan

Intermittent Fasting and Lifespan

If you limit the number of calories you consume, you will add more years to your lifespan. Remember that there is no pill you can take, no specific food you can consume, and there is no amount of exercise you can do actually to increase your longevity. What you need to do is to reduce the amount of food you consume, and your lifespan will increase.

How does it work? It happens that when you restrict the number of calories you consume, it will delay the onset of several age-related disorders such as diabetes, heart complications, cancer, and hypertension. Several types of research have found that there are lots of benefits that will accrue when you opt for intermittent fasting and calorie intake. Therefore you will experience;

- Reduced triglycerides

- Reduced inflammation.

- Reduced LDL

- Reduced blood pressure

- It will reduce the risk of cancer

- Increases HDL

- Increased fat loss and fat burning

- Improved body composition.

Intermittent fasting is all the rage in the modern world. You can see everything from the conservative 5:2 meal plan to more extremely intermittent fasting methods gaining popularity in the Silicon Valley circles. There has been lots of observational study pointing out the relationship between the intermittent fasting and the positive health effects.

New research from the Harvard University scientists has found that intermittent fasting slow aging, increase lifespan and promote your health by altering the activity of mitochondria networks inside your cells.

Mitochondria is a little like tiny power plant inside your cells. Recently a team of scientists that was led by Newcastle University showed how mitochondria are essential to the aging of cells. This new study from Harvard University showed how the change in the shapes of mitochondria networks affects your lifespan and your longevity. Also, the research showed how intermittent fasting could manipulate mitochondria networks so that it can keep them in a youthful state.

Generally, inside your mitochondria cell networks, two states alternate. One state is known as the fragmented state, and the other one is known as the fused state. They are using an organism, nematode worms, a species that is useful in studying longevity. The research found that restricted meals promote homeostasis in the mitochondria networks which allow for healthy plasticity between the fragmented and the fused states.

The study showed how essential is the plasticity of mitochondrial networks is the useful benefits of intermittent fasting. If you block mitochondrial in one state, you completely block the effects of intermittent fasting or the meal restriction on the longevity.

The research also showed that intermittent fasting enhances

the coordination of mitochondria with the peroxisomes. This is a type of organ that can be responsible for the increase of fatty acids oxidation. That is an essential fat metabolism process.

In the research experiments, the lifespan of the worms was witnessed to increase by simply the preservation of the mitochondria networks homeostasis through the dietary intervention. The study and the findings help us shed light on how intermittent fasting can increase your lifespan, and it can promote healthy aging.

Mitochondria are structures that produce energy in the cells. To protect them from external harm they fuse, and therefore they keep themselves in a more youthful state.

When the researchers restricted the worms from dieting, they found that the worms could keep their mitochondria in a fused state for an extended period. A similar result was achieved by the genetic manipulation of an energy protein known as AMP-activated protein kinase.

Researchers found that those youthful networks of mitochondria can increase the lifespan by communicating with the cellular structures known as organelles, that is peroxisomes, which are responsible for the control of metabolism.

Initially, researchers were not clear on how mitochondria fusion could affect the metabolism and the cellular function. The Harvard study showed that there is a relationship between the two and this results in an increased lifespan.

Previously low energy conditions such as intermittent fasting and dietary restriction have been proven to promote healthy aging.

The researchers believe that these findings will help them to develop strategies that can reduce the chances of developing age-related disorders as you get older. They are now investigating whether the same relationship is seen in mammals. They want to find whether mitochondria flexibility can reveal a correlation between obesity and some age-related disorders.

Chapter Fourteen: If And Exercises

What Does Exercise Look During Intermittent Fasting?

This depends on some factors starting from the type of intermittent fasting you choose. Some women fast for about 16 hours and eat for eight hours daily, while others may opt to eat between 500 and 600 calories on two nonconsecutive days per week to see how their body responds to it.

When it comes to intermittent fasting and exercises, it is good to listen to your body. If you feel too weak to do an extreme workout during intermittent fasting, you should take care of your diet and consider working out later.

While you should always give safety a priority, several techniques are perfect components to intermittent fasting.

Plan Your Meals around Your Workouts

Knowing that you are going to perform some exercises, then you should think about what food to eat the day before. This will significantly depend on the intensity of your workout. For instance, if you wish to build your glycogen stores with some complex carbohydrate for your dinner the day before so that you can have readily available energy for a cardio workout, then you should not do cardio on a full stomach. This is because the sudden demand of flow of the blood from the body muscles will use the required vital blood by your digestive system and in the assimilation of macronutrients.

What is most important here is to plan ahead of time so that your meal can meet the essential demands required by the workout intensity, even when it is the next day.

Which Workouts to Choose?

Not unless you find yourself lightheaded during fasting, do exercise to your heart's desire. This may range from weightlifting to cardio. Note that people tend to feel more focused when doing exercises and the more regularly they supplement fasting with exercises, the easier it gets and the more health benefits they derive from it.

If you have a carbohydrate centered meal to generate of energy, then you need to be more careful about some intense exercises like CrossFit especially towards the end of your fasting duration. This is because you may run out of energy and you may end up feeling nauseous, weak and lightheaded.

A less intense exercise during your intermittent fasting will allow your body to burn body fats to generate energy. This is a great idea if you are trying to trim some inches around your waist.

When to Back Off?

Note that in our previous section we have seen that when it comes to exercises and fasting, what is most important is to listen to your body. You will be at risk to do exercises on intermittent fasting if you have low body blood glucose.

Therefore if you are new to this diet, I would recommend a low-intensity class of exercises because you may faint or even pass out due to a decrease in the level of blood sugar in your body. You need to plan yourself so that you can go a long way.

What is important to consider when doing intermittent fasting from your dinner until your first meal the next day is what the type of your first meal of the day and how it fits in your exercise schedule. It is important to consume complex carbohydrates, plant-rich fibers, healthy fats, and proteins during the eating window so that you can maintain healthier intermittent fasting.

More plant fibers, more fats and more proteins are required on resting days while complex carbohydrates are needed during workout days.

So you have the message. Plan your diets accordingly, and more importantly, you should listen to your body.

Chapter Fifteen: If And Supplements

Your body requires a certain level of essential minerals and vitamins for survival. But this does not mean that you have to take them now and then. It does not imply that when you skip taking them in the morning, you are going to be severely deficient. Most of the vitamins and minerals are stored in your fat tissue, bones and other storage organs. The challenge is that if you are eating food several times a day, then you will be preventing your body from using those minerals. Your body stores as much back up of energy as it can, and this means that an abundant supply of nutrients that comes in will reduce your ability to use those minerals that are already stored in your body.

While you are doing intermittent fasting, your body breaks down all the dead cells and other waste materials that are already in your body. This process creates some energy, and it even gives you most of the macronutrients that you may require for short-term survival.

When you fast for longer periods, your body triggers autophagy, and metabolic pathways that helps your body to release micronutrients from mineral stores. Before that you will be getting enough nutrients from food given that you are eating non-processed foods.

Therefore you do not need to take lots of nutrients if you are eating a wide range of food. But there are some supplements you can take if you feel that you are deficient in some minerals and nutrients.

Another thing to point out is the use of supplements. And we will discuss how your body absorbs different minerals and vitamins.

Fat-soluble vitamins: These are vitamins that you need to take them with fats so that they can be absorbed easily. They include vitamin D, vitamin A, vitamin K and vitamin E. These fat-soluble vitamins are mostly stored in the body fat and in the liver. If you have decided to consume these supplements, then you need to combine them with real food that have some fat content in them. While doing intermittent fasting, you will be burning your body fats, and you can consider taking those vitamins that way.

Water-soluble vitamins: These vitamins aren't stored in your body, and they are excreted throughout the body if you are taking liquids. They include B- complex vitamins, vitamin C and folic acid. These vitamins are easily absorbed with pure water, and it is a good idea to take them more regularly if your diet is not that ready in vitamins.

But while fasting it is not necessary you supplement them not unless you are fasting for more than one week.

During Workouts

At this juncture, you are going to learn not only on how you can achieve your fat loss goals but also how you can optimize your performance while you are on an intermittent fasting diet.

To maximize your workout performance, it is good to train immediately before breaking your intermittent daily fasts and in doing that it will allow your body to replenish energy stores, protein synthesis and also to optimize recovery.

During the Day

Branched-chain Amino Acids: Human trials have been carried out, and it is estimated that sipping on branched chain amino acids when you are on intermittent fasting throughout the day may help to increase your protein synthesis. This help to balance out some of the protein breakdowns that may have occurred in your body.

Pre-workout

Caffeine: Caffeine does not only get you fired up, but it also increases the strength of your body.

Epigallocatechin – 3 Gallate: Remember that one of your primary goals of opting for intermittent fasting is to lose weight and therefore the essential goal of supplementation is to increase lipolysis and fatty acid oxidation.

Combining epigallocatechin – 3 – with caffeine leads to an increased metabolic change and fatty acid oxidation.

The combination of these two supplements may significantly boost the loss of weight while still minimizing any decrease in the rate of metabolism that may be observed during the periods of prolonged intermittent fasting. To increase your lipolysis, you need to take a dosage of about 150 milligrams of epigallocatechin - 3 – gallate per day.

But it may be much easier to ingest about 750 milligrams of green tea extracts that contain at least 30 percent of epigallocatechin – 3 gallates.

Beta-Alanine: This supplement increases the work capacity by simply decreasing fatigue that is associated with buildup of metabolites like hydrogen ions. Beta-alanine works by raising the level of carnosine which is an intracellular buffer that is stored in your body.

This buffer tends to reduce the acidity level in your blood to allow an improvement in high-intensity training performance. The recommended dosage of the beta-alanine supplement is approximately 4.5 grams per day.

Carbohydrates and Essential Amino Acids: Consuming about 35 grams of carbs and 6 grams of essential amino acids before a resistance exercise increases protein synthesis. This is caused by an increase in the influx of critical amino acids that activates your muscles.

This means that you need to consume about 100 grams of dried nuts and some essential amino acids before you hit the iron. This will help you to maximize your body muscle gains.

During Workout

Branched-chain amino acids: During resistance exercise, this supplement works in two ways. First, it helps to avoid a decrease in protein breakdown which results in enhanced recovery and secondly it decreases central fatigue by reducing the ratio of the branched chain amino acids to free tryptophan that is present in your blood.

Post Workout

Proteins: Consuming proteins after a resistance exercise may lead to an increase in the rate protein synthesis. Consumption of proteins immediately before and immediately after a resistance training leads to an increase in protein synthesis.

Carbohydrates: Immediately after a resistance training exercise consumption of carbs and an independent protein consumption leads to a decrease in muscle-protein catabolism with a slight increase in protein synthesis. Consuming carbohydrate immediately after a fasted training workout will help to restore your glycogen levels.

If you are opting for a post resistance training, then find the one that contains dextrose. This kind of resistance can restore glycogen at a higher rate than maltodextrin. If by any case you have decided to snack on actual food, then stick from moderate to high glycemic index food such as bananas, white rice, and potatoes.

Creatine: This supplement may lead to an increase in your lean body mass, strength, muscle fiber size, and power output. Therefore adding creatine supplement into your post resistance training workout schedule will help you to gain strength.

Chapter Sixteen: If And Hormones

Not only that, your body repairs and generates your essential organs and tissues while you are fasting and sleeping.

Intermittent fasting promises to improve your health and to reduce your body fats, but it holds up if only you do it consistently over an extended period. I believe you know that restricting the number of calories you eat can lead to the loss of weight in the short run.

The major challenge is the fact that only very few women will be willing to be on an intermittent fasting diet for their entire life. You need to note that more than 95 percent of women who lose weight by opting for the weight loss diets are always unable to sustain it and worse they end up in worse condition than they were.

Therefore while I want you to experience an immediate fat loss while still enhancing your health from adopting the intermittent fasting lifestyle, my major goal is for intermittent fasting to become a sustainable practice of your lifestyle so that you can experience the obvious benefits and long term results of intermittent fasting.

The good message is that you don't have to diet so that you can get the clear benefits of the intermittent fasting because you can enjoy most of your favorite meals when you do eat.

Intermittent Fasting for Women and Autophagy

In this section, I am going to explain in detail exactly how you can practice IFPC so that you can look and feel youthful regardless of your age. IFPC means that you alternate between the period's regular protein intake, protein restriction, and intermittent fasting. But it is important we understand not only how this method works but also why it works.

Before we dive into the details, you need to note that IFPC takes advantage of autophagy, in our previous chapters, I mentioned that autophagy is a biological term that was derived from the Greek autophagy. This Greek term has been translated to mean eating oneself. This is how your body cells clean themselves. They clean themselves by removing some waste products such as toxins from your body. This means that when your autophagy is functioning optimally, your body cells eat away at the junk, thereby recycling and removing the waste materials that could lead to the possible signs of aging.

The moment this process becomes impaired, and your body is continuously struggling to handle the problems, either from external or from the internal environment, waste materials can accumulate in your body tissues and cells. In turn, this can negatively affect the functioning of your body organs, and it will end up compromising your health.

As you get older, the autophagy becomes less efficient. Therefore it needs to be boosted so that your body cells can effectively and adequately remove their junk. How do you do this? The perfect way to do it is by taking a break from eating food for about 12 or even more hours. In doing this, you will allow your body's tissues and cells the time they require to clean themselves. At the same time, they will also switch their sources of energy from an external source of the meal to your body fats.

Intermittent fasting proteins cycling will provide an

alternating cyclic of nutrient deprivation and intake that can activate and influence the autophagy.

Intermittent fasting can do this by depriving your body cells of nutrients when you are fasting. Particularly it functions by activating the hormone glucagon. This hormone works in the opposite direction to insulin to keep your body blood sugar levels balanced. Imagine a balancing seesaw; if one side goes down, the other side goes up. Note that the moment you give your body macronutrients through the consumption of food, automatically the insulin level goes up and the glucagon hormone goes down. The reverse process will happen if you deny your body macronutrients, that is, glucagon will rise while the insulin will decrease.

What you need to keep in mind is that glucagon hormone triggers autophagy. That is the reason as to why if you withhold macronutrients by intermittent fasting it will boost the youth of your body cells.

The Frequency of Intermittent Fasting

The idea here is to cycle your intermittent fasting days. This means that you should fast only three non-consecutive days in a week. This will help to balance your hormones. Medical experts show that cycles of intermittent fasting can reduce the risk of cancer, decrease visceral fats, improve your immune system and to an extent increase your longevity. Most of the well-known benefits of intermittent fasting such as decreasing the risk of the development of heart diseases and diabetes can be attributed to the activation of autophagy.

Also protein, cycling has a similar effect on intermittent fasting. If you restrict protein consumption for short durations of time, it will help you to keep autophagy working correctly and efficiently. Protein cycling does work to enhance youthfulness because your body cells can't create its proteins. Instead, protein restriction accelerates your body to recycle the existing proteins you have already provided it. For most women, they do not normally deprive themselves of proteins. But scientists indicate that there is a clear relationship between the cellular control process of autophagy and the protein intake.

What is most important is that this process of autophagy is required to maintain your muscle mass. In an experiment when the autophagy process was intentionally prevented in rats, their muscles atrophied, and they were seen to become weak. But this is not surprising since you know the essential of sleeping to your muscle growth. For most women autophagy process is high when they are sleeping.

Restricting protein consumption for about eight hours per day in a cyclic pattern can be beneficial to women. In addition to enhancing your autophagy, there is clear evidence that protein cycling can help to reduce the risk of heart diseases, cancer and diabetes especially in women who are under the age of sixty-five.

How Intermittent Fasting Protein Cycling Works

You will have to choose three non- consecutive low days that are intended to activate the autophagy in your body. Here you will starve your body cells of macronutrients along with the remaining four high days to inhibit autophagy.

During your low days, you should fast overnight then you limit your protein consumption for the remaining 8 hours of the day. During this period and time, you should aim at eating less than 25 grams of proteins. During your high days, you will not restrict food item consumption.

IFPC is purposely intended in this alternating cyclic of inhibition and activation. This is essential since the low intake is not always good because you can't live in a constant state of macronutrient deprivation. Also, too much of protein restriction can contribute to the aging in the form of muscle wasting that is accompanied by an increase in immunity deficiencies and weakness.

To ensure sure that you reap the benefits of protein restriction and intermittent fasting in a healthy way for a woman's body, the cyclical combination of high days, low days and intermittent fasting is essential to the practice of IFPC.

You may select any day of the week to be either high or low, but you need to keep in mind that the three low days must be non-consecutive.

Here's what your typical week of IFPC may appear:

- **Sunday**: High – no food item limitations

- **Monday**: Low – Fast for 16 hours, then consume low-protein for 8 hours

- **Tuesday**: High – no food item restrictions

- **Wednesday**: Low – Fast for 16 hours, then consume low protein for 8 hours

- **Thursday**: High – no food restrictions

- **Friday**: Low – Fast for 16 hours, then consume low protein for 8 hours

- **Saturday**: High – no food restrictions

The best part about IFPC is that it works better when customized for your life. For instance, if you hate skipping breakfast, then you can start your fast earlier the night before so that you can get your full 16 hours and you will still have your morning diet. Are you craving for a slice of a burger? Then go for it. But understand that you will only have approximately 5 grams of proteins remaining before hitting your daily limit. The choice lies with you. You are the only person with the power to feel and look younger. You need to remember that with IFPC the low and high can give you a fantastic, long-lasting glow.

Intermittent Fasting and Female Hormones

In your entire life decisions, experimenting with intermittent fasting may seem tiny. But unfortunately for some ladies, it appears that tiny decisions can have severe impacts on their health either positive or negative.

It appears that the hormonal regulating vital functions, for instance, ovulation, are susceptible to your energy consumption.

In women, hypothalamic pituitary gonadal axis, which is the cooperative functioning of 3 endocrine glands acts like an air traffic controller.

To start, the hypothalamus will release gonadotropin-releasing hormone. This then directs the pituitary to release a hormone known as luteinizing hormone and another hormone known as the follicular stimulating hormone.

Later the luteinizing and follicular stimulating hormones act on the gonads, that is ovaries. This is what triggers the production of progesterone and estrogen in women. These hormones are essential because they help you to release mature eggs. They also help to support your pregnancy.

Now because this chain of reactions happens typically on a specific and regular cycle in women, gonadotropin-releasing hormone pulses should be precisely timed, or otherwise, everything will go out of control.

Gonadotropin-releasing hormone is very sensitive to some environmental factors, and it can be thrown off by intermittent fasting. It is important to note that even short-term intermittent fasting, for instance, three days are worse enough to alter hormonal pulses in a group of some women.

There is even evidence that even missing a single regular diet can put you on alert, thereby perking up your antennae, so your body is ready to respond to the unexpected change in the energy intake

That can be a good reason as to why some women do well with intermittent fasting while others run into deep problems.

Why does Intermittent Fasting affect Women's Hormones?

The whole issue has something to do with the kisspeptin. Kisspeptin is a protein like a molecule that helps neurons to communicate with each other.

Kisspeptin is responsible for the stimulation of gonadotropin-releasing hormone production in women, and it is susceptible to insulin, ghrelin and leptin hormones that tend to react to satiety and hunger.

What you need to note is that women have more amount of kisspeptin protein as compared to men. This means greater sensitivity to slight changes in energy balance.

Therefore this is one of the major reasons why intermittent fasting causes the production of women's kisspeptin to dip, tossing their gonadotropin-releasing hormone off kilter.

Fertility, Meet Metabolism

I know you are asking yourself; what are the effects if the kisspeptin protein drops and I miss monthly periods? Am I going to have kids?

Here is the explanation.

The female metabolism and reproductive systems are deeply intertwined. Note that if you are missing monthly periods, it means that a bunch of your hormones has negatively ben affected and not just the pregnancy hormones.

In general terms, women tend to consume fewer proteins, and therefore fasting women will even take fewer proteins. Consuming fewer proteins implies that you are consuming fewer amino acids.

Why are amino acids so important to the health of a woman? They are essential because they are required to activate estrogen receptors and to synthesize insulin growth factor in the liver. The insulin growth factor is responsible for triggering the uterine wall lining to thicken and the progression of the reproduction cycle.

Therefore low protein meals can reduce women's fertility.

You have estrogen receptors throughout your body including in your brains, bones and GI tract. When you change estrogen balance in your body, you change metabolic function all over your body. This may include but not limited to digestion, protein turnover, recovery, bone formation, cognition, and moods.

On matters to do with energy balance and appetite, estrogen hormone works in several ways.

First and foremost, in your brainstem, estrogen modifies the peptides that signal you to feel hungry (ghrelin) or full (cholecystokinin).

Secondly, in the hypothalamus, estrogen hormones stimulate neurons that trigger the production of appetite-regulating peptides.

If you do something that will cause your estrogen hormone to drop, you will find yourself feeling hungrier and eating lots more as you would do under normal situations.

Estrogen hormones are therefore the critical metabolic regulators. This is because of the ratios of estrogen metabolites, that is, estradiol, estrone and estriol change over time. Note that before your menopause, estradiol is the dominant player in the game, but after the menopause, its level decreases while the concentration of estrone remains about the same.

It is essential to note that the duties of each and estrogen remain unclear, though some theories explain that a decrease in estradiol estrogen may lead to an increase it fats storage. This is because fats are used to make estradiol.

This explains why most women find it harder to lose some fats after menopause. This should serve as a key reason as to why you should be concerned about your reproductive system and health even if you may not be focusing on making babies.

Low energy meals reduce the fertility of some women. If you are too lean, it becomes a disadvantage to your reproductive system. A female body is exquisitely tuned to any threat to her energy and fertility.

Thinking about it critically, it makes sense.

Women are unique species in the world of mammals. Note that almost all other mammals can pause or terminate a pregnancy pretty more natural whenever they wish to do so, but female humans cannot do that.

In female humans, the placenta tends to breach the maternal blood vessels, and therefore the fetus takes the control.

The baby inside a woman can block the action of insulin hormone to hoard more sugar for itself. Moreover, the fetus can make the blood vessels of the mother to dilate thereby adjusting the blood pressure so that it can get more nutrients.

You should bear in your mind that the baby is always determined to survive no matter how much it will cost the mother. This phenomenon is referred to as maternal-fetal conflict and scientists compare it to the host-virus relationship.

Once you are pregnant, you cannot sweet talk your fetus to stop developing and growing. It could be fatal during the famine. This is the reason as to why your reproductive system is much sensitive to metabolic cues at several levels.

How Does your Body Know?

Note that your hormonal balance is specifically sensitive to how often, how much and what you eat.

But how does your body realize when food is insufficiency?

For many decades people used to believe that it was the

percentage of fats in a woman body that regulated their reproductive system.

Their idea was if a woman fat reserve dropped below a certain percentage, that is 11 %, hormones would be messed up and her monthly period would stop.

This makes lots of sense since if there is not much food to eat, you will automatically lose weight over time. But note that the situation may be worse than that. The availability of food may change very quickly. I believe you are aware that if you have ever tried to lose some weight, your body fats often took a while to drop even if you were consuming fewer calories.

Therefore women who are not lean can stop ovulating and even lose their monthly periods.

That is why overall energy balance is more critical to this process than your body fats percentage.

Energy Balance and Stressors

Particularly, negative energy balance in most women may be to be blamed for the hormonal domino effect, and it is not just about how much food you consume. Negative energy balance can be caused by consuming too little food, too many exercises, poor nutrition, too much stress, too little rest, and chronic inflammation.

Any combination of those stressors can put you into negative energy balance, and you can stop ovulating: nursing the flu and training for a marathon; fewer vegetables and fruits; intermittent fasting and too much stress.

Your body cannot tell the distinction between something

imaginary and a real threat that may be generated by your feelings and thoughts.

Cortisol, which is a stress hormone inhibits your GnRH, and it suppresses your ovaries production of progesterone and estrogen hormones.

During stress, the progesterone hormone is converted to cortisol hormone, and therefore more cortisol implies less progesterone. This is what causes estrogen hormone to dominate in the HPG axis which is a severe problem.

Your body could be having about 30% of fats but when your energy balance is negatively affected especially during intermittent fasting your reproduction may stop.

What Should You Do?

Based on what I have explained in the previous section, intermittent fasting may affect your reproductive health. This is possible if your body sees intermittent fasting as a significant stressor.

Note that anything that negatively affects your reproductive system affects your general health and your fitness.

Intermittent fasting protocols vary with some being more extreme than others. Factors such as your nutritional status, the duration of fasting and your age are likely relevant.

So is Intermittent Fasting Yours?

Bearing in mind how much remains unclear, I would suggest you start with a conservative approach.

Therefore if you want to try intermittent fasting, it is a good idea to start with a gentle protocol and pay more attention to how things will behave.

When to Stop Intermittent Fasting?

You should stop intermittent fasting if:

- Your hair falls out

- When you start developing dry skin

- When your monthly periods become irregular or stops

- When you start experiencing challenges staying asleep

- Your injuries are not healing quickly

- When your moods start to swing

- When your tolerance to stress decreases

- When you realize that you are not recovering from workouts easily

- When your interest in romance decreases and your lady sexual parts are not responding to it when it happens.

- When you notice that your digestion is slowing down

- When you start feeling cold.

Never try Intermittent Fasting if:

The fact of the matter is that intermittent fasting is not for every woman, and you should not bother experimenting with it if;

- If you do not sleep well

- If you are pregnant

- If you are in chronic stress

- If you are new to exercise and diet

Pregnant women need a lot of energy. Therefore if you are starting a family, intermittent fasting is not a perfect idea.

If you are under stress or maybe you are experiencing challenges with your sleep, then your body requires to be nurtured but not additional stress.

If in the previous periods you have experienced eating disorders, then intermittent fasting could lead you to chronic complications.

You do not need to mess with your health with intermittent fasting. You can achieve similar benefits by opting to other diets.

If you are new to exercise and diet, then intermittent fasting may appear like a magic bullet for the loss of weight.

It would be a wise decision you address any nutritional deficiency before you can consider experimenting with intermittent fasting. Therefore you need to ensure that you start from a strong or solid nutritional foundation.

What to do if Intermittent Fasting is not for you

How can you lose weight and get your desired shape if intermittent fasting is not the perfect option for you? It is straightforward.

You need to learn the essentials of good nutritional diets. This is the best thing you can do for your overall health and fitness.

Cook and eat whole food. Do exercises more regularly and stay consistent.

It is true that intermittent fasting is a popular diet in the modern world. And maybe your husband, your boyfriend or your brother finds it as an excellent tool for good health and fitness.

But you should remember that women bodies are very different from those of men.

Frequently Asked Questions

What is Intermittent Fasting?

Intermittent fasting is an eating plan where you cycle between periods of eating and not eating food. There are several kinds of intermittent fasting, but all of them serve the same purpose. They give your body time to operate without food--16-24 hours-- so that your body can spend most of its energy on internal repair and healing. Sometimes this cannot happen when you are always in a feeding state.

Who is Intermittent Fasting Meant for?

Based on its numerous health benefits, intermittent fasting is for everyone who is serious about improving his or her overall health and losing some pounds of weight without necessarily overhauling their diet.

Generally, you do not have to change anything about your meal plan so that you can benefit from intermittent fasting and this makes it more appealing to many women.

It is also meant to those who want to burn extra fat while still maintaining their body muscles.

This diet is entirely safe to opt, and it provides several benefits, and therefore it is a matter of committing to it and seeing if it is a diet you want to adopt more regularly.

What are the Benefits of Intermittent Fasting?

There are several benefits of intermittent fasting. And if you are wondering how to do intermittent fasting to get these benefits, check the below benefits and all are backed by evidence.

1. Increased Life Span

Studies on animals are being carried out by Dr. Mattson Mark and his colleagues at the National Institute of Aging. Their findings from these researches are that animals tend to age slower and live for an extended period when they consume a fewer number of calories. Their research shows that this effect can only be achieved by consuming less food daily or by opting for intermittent fasting.

1. Improvement in Hormone Profile

When you fast, you get significant reductions in insulin and blood sugar levels. It also leads to an increase in your growth hormone. All these are favorable for maintaining muscle, losing weight, reduced risk of insulin resistance, heart and diabetes disorders.

2. Fast Weight Loss

Most women want to do intermittent fasting because they have heard that intermittent fasting is an effective and safe way to lose weight. And they are correct.

Several types of research have shown that both obese and overweight subjects burn more fats and lose significant pounds of weight with intermittent fasting.

Other benefits of intermittent fasting include;

1. An increase in lipolysis and fat oxidation

2. A decrease in the levels of blood sugar

3. Leads to the maintenance of your skeletal muscle mass

4. Can lead to an increase in insulin sensitivity and a decrease in insulin levels

5. Increases epinephrine and norepinephrine levels which increase fats breakdown.

6. An increase in the levels of glucagon which breaks down body fats

7. An increase in the levels of the growth hormone which helps to preserve muscle mass.

Why is Intermittent Fasting Effective?

2014 review of the literature indicated that intermittent fasting's power comes typically from its impact on the adaptive cellular response that reduces oxidative damage & inflammation, improves cellular production and optimizes energy metabolism.

The review showed that intermittent fasting was able to protect rodents against cancers, diabetes, neurodegeneration, and heart diseases while in female humans intermittent fasting help to reduce hypertension, obesity, rheumatoid and asthma.

An earlier review that was conducted back in the year 2005 and published in the journal entitled Nutritional Biochemistry indicated that the health benefits of intermittent fasting come as a result of at least two mechanisms: an increase in cellular stress resistance and a reduction in oxidative damage.

Generally, that implies that intermittent fasting helps your body to deal with stress including coping with fasting which is also a form of stress by itself.

Intermittent fasting also triggers the autophagy process which tends to break down, and it recycles cellular debris and dysfunctional proteins.

This process is similar to cleaning up around your house, a process you would hope to take place in your body on a regular basis.

I believe that this has given you an understanding of how intermittent fasting works magic in your body cells.

Why Does Intermittent Fasting Burn Body Fats?

Earlier I listed some intermittent fasting benefits, and most of the benefits are centered around fat loss.

Here is a summary plus some mechanism through which intermittent fasting increases fat burning in your body.

- An increase in uncoupling protein – 3 mRNA which is essential for the production of energy in your body cells.

- An increase in the levels of epinephrine and norepinephrine which accelerates fat breakdown.

- An increase in the levels of glucagon which breaks down your body fats.

- An increase in the levels of growth hormones which preserves your body muscle mass and thus leading to a healthy metabolic rate which in turn burns body fat.

- Increased activation of a sensitive lipase hormone.

Generally, when you go for an extended period without eating, you direct your body to rely on the stored fats. This is a similar process that is being experienced with extreme and consistent exercise training.

Your body understands that to maintain blood glucose and the stored carbohydrates for the possible immediate use; it is better to rely on fats which provide more energy, that is about nine calories per one gram as compared to protein or carbohydrates that has four calories per one gram.

How to do and When to Begin Intermittent Fasting?

For women, the benefits of intermittent fasting are too many to ignore. So where will you start?

It should not be so awful. There is an approach that makes intermittent fasting doable and straightforward. The procedure is a bit of a cheat, but you need to note that it does not lessen its benefits. Therefore you should give it a try.

The day before your 1st day fast should your 1st feast. During that, three hours after you have enjoyed your last meal of for that day, you should start your timer on your 1st day fast.

For instance, if you enjoyed your dinner at around 6 p.m, your body will be in a semi-fasted state at around 9 pm. You need to consider that as the kickoff of your fasting. Hit the sack and consider sleeping for 8 hours. By the time you will be waking up, you will have completed a 3rd of your day's fasting without eating anything.

You may not feel hungry when you wake up in the morning. This will depend on the amount of food that you consumed the day before. For breakfast, you can keep yourself energized by taking lots of water, and wait until lunchtime. If you do a simple calculation, you will have knocked out about 14 hours of your fasting. And if you are strong to make it to at least 3 pm, then you will have fasted for 18 good hours.

At this point, you may be really on fire. You can take a glass of peppermint tea to reward yourself. This is when the tons of health benefits from your short-term fasting will start kicking in.

At this juncture, if you really cannot help it, you can consume a small meal or smoothies to break your fasting. But if you want to win, then you need to power through to dinner without eating anything. The moment you reach 9 pm, you will have made it. You will have completed your fasting, and you can retire to bed thinking about your breakfast.

If you cannot wait until the following day morning to eat, it is advisable you take a meal with a high level of protein. You can shake it with a few carbohydrates about two hours before you sleep. In doing that, you will be providing your muscles with essential proteins while keeping your belly fully satisfied until morning.

The 1st day fast is not easy, but at the same time it is possible, and when you stay focused on the benefits of intermittent fasting it becomes simple and doable. It is something you can do.

What makes intermittent fasting easier is by deciding to do it. Most women have experienced tough times when they do fasting because they constantly think what they will be eating next after the periods of fasting. That feels too much for them to handle.

When you consciously make a firm decision that tomorrow will be a fasting day, you activate a new mechanism in your body. You will be forcing innards to recharge while you reflect on the poor consumption habits with which you have been self-medicating. Intermittent fasting is such an important tool for deep change, and that is the reason as to why most women around the world have been turning to it.

That is all you need to consider starting your intermittent fasting.

How to do Intermittent Fasting for the Loss of Weight?

It is similar to what I have explained above. The simple and the easiest way to do intermittent fasting for the loss of weight is to do it once in a week.

Although several studies on intermittent fasting have considered alternate day fasting as the best, it looks a bit crazy. You can lose fats and weight with just opting for a single day of fasting each week.

Therefore, you should finish consuming your dinner and start your fasting after that. If you are strong enough to make it to the next day's dinner, then you stand a chance to win on your journey to weight loss. Note that when you are in a fasted state, your body relies on its fat stores to generate energy.

Therefore it helps your body to burn fat instead of glucose. It is a very freeing process.

What Should I Consume after Intermittent Fasting?

Among the essential steps in learning how to do intermittent fasting to figure out how you can ease the process of going back into eating.

The moment you finish your fasting you should pretend as if you never fasted. This means that you do not have to reward or compensate yourself in a special way of eating.

Once you decide to stop fasting, you need to forget about it and consume food the exact way you would do at the particular time of the day. What you need to do is to eat responsibly.

This implies that if you end your fasting at lunchtime, have lunch. For instance, if you end your fasting at 12:00 pm and you do not typically have lunch until 2:00 or 3: pm, then you should have a sort of light snacks, but it should not be large than what you would typically consume at that time.

Note that there is no special way to end your fasting. The best thing you should do is to pretend that you never fasted and begin consuming food in the exact way you would do at that particular time of the day.

Many women tend to crave for healthier food at the end of their fasting. As a result, they end up selecting healthy snacks or green smoothies instead of devouring large pizzas as you may think would happen after long hours of not eating anything.

Is Intermittent Fasting Good or Bad for my Blood Sugar?

The truth of the matter is that low body blood sugar is not common as most women believe. But you need to check with your professional doctor in case you are not certain.

A large group of healthy women population can maintain body blood sugars levels that are not too low nor too high in a whole range of different circumstances including intense exercise and intermittent fasting.

In a study that examined the effects of 24 hours fasting, it was concluded that fasting didn't cause the levels of body blood glucose to go below 3.5 mmol per liter. This means that during the 24 hours fasting body blood sugar gradually lowered itself, but it remained at normal non-hypoglycemic levels.

Can I do Exercises when on Intermittent Fasting?

I recommend you perform as many exercises as you can during intermittent fasting. In any health nutrition, exercises are fundamental and therefore intermittent fasting diet is not an exemption. Both mountain biking and yoga are excellent exercises that can complement intermittent fasting.

Given that you are performing resistance exercises at least three times a week, then you will not lose muscles because intermittent fasting increases your growth hormones which help to preserve your muscles.

What you will notice when you do extensive workouts on the day that you are fasting, your levels of energy will go down.

The reason to that is because the workouts will be using the lowered glycogen reserves and this implies you may experience fatigue more sooner than on a normal or a traditional eating day.

What you need to understand is that doing exercises for short durations at high intensity when your body is on a fasted state is the perfect weapon. I, therefore, encourage you to explore them as it will boost fat loss in your body.

Why do I Feel Hungry when Intermittent Fasting?

Your belly might experience hunger because you are not consuming any food during intermittent fasting.

In addition to that, the ghrelin which is your hunger hormone may respond to a lack of food in your stomach, and this triggers your brain to think that you are starving.

Generally, hunger pangs after about three fasts as your body adjusts.

Why do I Experience Headaches when Intermittent Fasting?

Remember that it is not everyone who experiences that. But it has been proven that most Muslim women on Ramadan fasting experience headaches. It appears that most women are susceptible to headaches while intermittent fasting.

This may not be due to dehydration as you may think, and it may even be due to withdrawal symptoms. It is similar to what you may experience when you quit taking a coffee cold turkey.

If you experience headaches at the beginning of your fasting, it will go away after some fasting.

If the situation gets worse, you should treat your headaches as you normally would do when not fasting. But more importantly, drink tons of water and get fresh air during your intermittent fasting.

Can I Drink anything During Intermittent Fasting?

You can drink but make sure that what you drink is free of calories. This does not mean that you take any drink. For instance, drinking diet soda is not okay. You need to drink herbal tea and tons of water.

Some women think that drinking black coffee when intermittent fasting is okay, but I will not advise you to drink it. Generally, the caffeine that is present in the coffee may skyrocket your epinephrine which in turn may assist you to lose weight, but since I discourage you from drinking coffee, in general, you better do away with it especially when its caffeine it is buffered by food.

Instead of drinking coffee, you need to focus on drinking tons of water or herbal teas that you enjoy without adding milk or sugar. Remember that should be a rest day for your body, and this means that you should not take calories of any kind.

Can I Take Supplements When Intermittent Fasting?

You can take supplements, but it is good to give your body a break. Therefore if you are taking probiotics, fish oil or multivitamins, then take a day off from supplements.

This will prevent your body from developing sensitivities to commonly consumes ingredients and supplements that could occur with the continued consumption of any food item.

How Regularly Should I do Intermittent Fasting?

Generally, this depends on the type of intermittent fasting that you opt, but if you decide to follow my 1-day fasting schedule, then once in a week is perfect. Some women decide to do two 24 hours intermittent fasts in a week, and they have seen outstanding results doing so, but this should on the higher end.

Why do I Feel cold When Intermittent Fasting?

Intermittent fasting increases the flow of the blood to your body fat a process known as adipose tissue blood flow.

This means that when you are doing intermittent fasting, more blood flows to your body fat so that it can move it to your body muscles where it is burned to generate energy. Due to the increased flow to your body fat, vasoconstriction may occur in your fingertips and even in your toes to compensate.

Does Intermittent Fasting Slow Down Metabolism?

Most women despite all the benefits intermittent fasting still wonder whether it will slow down their metabolism to a halt. Maybe you have been advised to consume food after every 2 hours, or otherwise, your metabolism will slow down, and you will end up storing fats in your body. That could not be the truth.

Back in the year 2000, in a research that was published in the American Journal of Clinical Nutrition, the participants went through four days of intermittent fasting. The research aimed to determine the effect on their resting energy expenditure. This is the amount of energy that your body requires to perform all of its basic functions and operations when you are resting.

The outcome may surprise you because, for the first three days, all the participants saw metabolism or resting energy expenditure increase!

In another similar research by a different group of scientists, the participants who opted for alternate day fasting for about 22 days did not experience any decrease in their rate of metabolism.

Moreover, women who were on resistance exercise programs and low-calorie meals did not experience any decrease in their resting metabolic rate, and these participants were only consuming 800 calories per day for 12 weeks.

In other studies, there was no change in the metabolic rates of women who opted to skip breakfast or who opted for only two meals a day as compared to six meals per day.

What you should notice therefore is that food or lack of food in the short-term has nothing to do with your metabolic rate.

Your metabolic rate is more closely tied to your weight especially your body muscle mass. This means that when your body fat goes down or up, so does your metabolic rate changes.

Therefore, short-term intermittent fasting can provide you with incredible benefits without sabotaging your metabolism rate.

You do not need to be scared about your metabolism and your intermittent fasting. Intermittent fasting has no negative impacts on your metabolic rate.

Is Intermittent Fasting Safe for all Women?

This is the biggest area of concentration when discussing intermittent fasting. Most people caution women against opting to intermittent fasting because it affects their fertility.

That may be true but what many people fail to understand is that all of this information is based on alternate day intermittent fasting where women are typically not consuming anything every other day.

That is why women hormones are messed up leading to fertility issues.

Therefore one-day fasting per week is the best for all women because it is safer.

There is research that looked at the impact of short-term intermittent fasting on the monthly period of women. The study concluded that, despite the metabolic changes that may occur during intermittent fasting, even fasting for long hours like 72 hours do not affect the menstrual cycle of a normal and healthy woman.

In addition to that even more, extended fasting has little impact on the monthly menstrual periods of normal women.

But other studies suggest that longer fasts that are more than 72 hours may affect the monthly period of some lean women whose their fat levels are below 20 percent.

Generally, intermittent fasting is safe for women. It is effective, safe and a healthy way of burning fat in women to give them shapes and sizes.

Does it take long to get into Ketosis state?

Generally, it can take anywhere between twelve and twenty-four hours to get into a partial ketosis state. During intermittent fasting, the moment your serum sugar level decreases by 20 percent, your liver starts to produce ketones that are used to supplement the energy that your brains require.

To achieve full ketosis can take even up to ten days. Upon entering ketosis, some women will experience a sort of a fruity smell when they are breathing, lethargy or a decrease in appetite, while some women do not experience these symptoms at all. If you want to remain in full ketosis for a long duration, you should consume fewer calories, that is, less than thirty grams of carbs each day.

However, the metabolic benefits of fasting do not depend on achieving your full ketosis state while doing intermittent fasting. Your resistance level can decrease to about 40 percent if you stick to intermittent fasting for just a few weeks.

Conclusion

I believe you have read useful information in this book. You have learned how intermittent fasting can change your way of living. What you need to remember is that intermittent fasting has lots of benefits.

Intermittent fasting has gained popularity for the past few decades with many discussions surrounding it. The majority of women, especially in the western nations, are opting for this diet. It has been proven to improve the health of women. For instance, it can reduce the risk of cancer and diabetes in women.

To succeed in your intermittent fasting journey, you need to follow this ultimate guide. The content contained in this book has been thoroughly researched, and most of the conclusions are drawn out of medical expert findings and from practical experience.